# Nursing Professional Development Competencies

## TOOLS TO EVALUATE AND ENHANCE EDUCATIONAL PRACTICE

*Barbara A. Brunt, MA, MN, RN-BC, NE-BC, FABC*

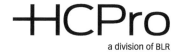

HCPro

a division of BLR

*Nursing Professional Development Competencies: Tools to Evaluate and Enhance Educational Practice* is published by HCPro, a division of BLR

Download the additional materials of this book at *www.hcpro.com/downloads/12244.*

ISBN: 978-1-55645-079-2

HCPro provides information resources for the healthcare industry.

*MAGNET™, MAGNET RECOGNITION PROGRAM®, and ANCC MAGNET RECOGNITION® are trademarks of the American Nurses Credentialing Center (ANCC). The products and services of HCPro, a division of BLR, are neither sponsored nor endorsed by the ANCC. The acronym "MRP" is not a trademark of HCPro or its parent company.

HCPro is not affiliated in any way with The Joint Commission, which owns the JCAHO and Joint Commission trademarks.

Barbara A. Brunt, MA, MN, RN-BC, NE-BC, FABC

Julia W. Aucoin, DNS, RN-BC, CNE

Elizabeth Petersen, Vice President

Vincent Skyers, Design Manager

Michael McCalip, Layout/Graphic Design

Rebecca Hendren, Product Manager

Erin Callahan, Senior Director, Product

Matt Sharpe, Production Supervisor

Vicki McMahan, Senior Graphic Designer

Tyson Davis, Cover Designer

Advice given is general. Readers should consult professional counsel for specific legal, ethical, or clinical questions.

Arrangements can be made for quantity discounts. For more information, contact:

HCPro

75 Sylvan Street, Suite A-101

Danvers, MA 01923

Telephone: 800-650-6787 or 781-639-1872

Fax: 800-639-8511

Email: *customerservice@hcpro.com*

Visit HCPro online at

*www.hcpro.com* and *www.hcmarketplace.com*

# Table of Contents

Dedication ..........................................................................................................................vii

About the Author ........................................................................................................... ix

Acknowledgments ......................................................................................................... xi

About This Book ............................................................................................................ xiii

List of Figures ................................................................................................................xv

Introduction ..................................................................................................................xv

**Section I: Competency Assessment and Validation** ...................................................1

Chapter 1: Overview of the Competency Movement ..................................................... 3

Key Concepts.................................................................................................................3

Why Is Competence Important?....................................................................................4

What Is Competence in Nursing?..................................................................................4

Competency-Based Education .....................................................................................5

Evidence-Based Practice and Practice-Based Evidence................................................7

Competencies for Nursing Professional Development Specialists ................................9

Difference Between NPD Competencies and Academic Educator Competencies ..........9

Chapter 2: Developing Educator Competencies............................................................13

Performing a Nursing Professional Development Research Study ................................13

Origins of the Competencies .......................................................................................14

Ongoing Research .......................................................................................................15

Validating the Results ..................................................................................................15

Refining the Results .....................................................................................................16

Additional Research......................................................................................................16

Chapter 3: Additional Competencies Based on Revised Standards...............................19

Additional Competencies .............................................................................................19

Technology....................................................................................................................21

EBP and PBE ................................................................................................................22

Excellence Initiatives.....................................................................................................24

Transformational Leadership ...............................................................25

Career Development and Role Transition .................................................27

Peer Review .......................................................................................28

Emotional Intelligence .........................................................................29

## Chapter 4: Benner's Novice-to-Expert Continuum ..........................31

Dreyfus Model of Skill Acquisition..........................................................32

Educating Nurses................................................................................35

Applications of Benner's Theory.............................................................36

## Chapter 5: Creating a Framework for Educator Competencies.............41

Framework .........................................................................................42

NPD Specialist Practice Model ..............................................................43

What Was Done ..................................................................................44

Final List of Competencies by Category ..................................................45

## Chapter 6: Methods to Validate Competencies ...............................49

How Do You Measure Competence? .......................................................49

Competency Checklists ........................................................................50

Other Tools to Validate Competence ......................................................51

Competencies and Performance .............................................................53

Differentiating Levels of Competence......................................................54

# Section II: Applications of the Competencies to Practice .............. 57

## Chapter 7: Self-Assessment Tool....................................................59

Use as a Self-Assessment Tool ...............................................................59

## Chapter 8: Developing Criterion-Based Position Descriptions ............61

Criterion-Based Position Descriptions......................................................61

## Chapter 9: Orientations for New Educators .....................................79

Orientation for New Educators ..............................................................79

## Chapter 10: Performance Appraisals, Peer Review, and Professional
## Development Plans.........................................................................89

Using the Checklist for Yearly Performance Appraisals.................................89

Peer Review .......................................................................................92

Professional Development Plan...............................................................92

Reflect on Development........................................................................93

## Chapter 11: Creating a Professional Portfolio ..................................95

Why Create a Portfolio? .......................................................................95

Types of Portfolios ..............................................................................97

Building a Portfolio .............................................................................97

Helping Others Develop Professional Portfolios.........................................98

Use of Portfolios in Education ..................................................................................................99

## Chapter 12: Developing Cultural Competence ...............................................101

Cultural Competence and Nursing Professional Development Specialists..................................101

Barriers to Cultural Competence..............................................................................................103

Strategies to Promote Cultural Competence ............................................................................103

Research...................................................................................................................................104

## Chapter 13: Understanding Generational Differences ...................................107

Characteristics of the Various Generations...............................................................................107

Teaching Strategies with the Various Generations ....................................................................109

Strategies for Managers ..........................................................................................................112

Research...................................................................................................................................112

## Chapter 14: Applications of the Competencies..............................................115

Graduate Nursing Education Programs.....................................................................................115

Scope and Standards of Nursing Professional Development .....................................................116

Resource for Certification Exam ...............................................................................................116

Job Function Analysis ..............................................................................................................116

Development Plan for New Role ...............................................................................................117

ANCC Magnet Recognition Program® .....................................................................................117

Need for Additional Research ..................................................................................................117

## Chapter 15: Educational Implications of the Institute of Medicine Report...................119

NPD Specialist Role in Helping Meet IOM Recommendations...................................................120

Issues Relating to Education.....................................................................................................121

## Appendix ...................................................................................................123

# Dedication

The first edition of this book was dedicated to three individuals who have passed away, but who had a tremendous impact on my life. I want to acknowledge them in this edition also.

First I want to thank Doris Gosnell, my mentor, colleague, and friend. She decided to take a chance by hiring a nurse with an associate's degree in nursing and a bachelor's degree in education. When I first started my staff development career in 1978, I worked with nursing assistants and other non-professional staff. Through Doris's guidance and mentoring, I assumed more and more responsibility in that department, becoming a coordinator, and then ultimately the director of the department when she retired. She supported me as I went through my master's program in community health education, but always told me I needed to get a master's degree in nursing. I am sorry that she did not live to see me achieve that goal.

Next, I want to acknowledge my late husband, John G. Brunt. In our 34 years of marriage, he always supported my professional nursing endeavors, even though it took away from our time together. He was there as I completed the pilot and first four phases of the initial research study. I miss his smile, his sense of adventure, and his outgoing disposition.

Finally, I want to acknowledge my father, Raymond G. Johnson. As I worked for him at Johnson's Furniture throughout my junior high and high school years, I developed my work ethic and values, as well as my organizational and communication skills, which have served me well in my career path. He and Mom helped support me financially as I went through college and provided an ongoing source of encouragement throughout my life.

# About the Author

## Barbara A. Brunt, MA, MN, RN-BC, NE-BC, FABC

**Barbara A. Brunt, MA, MN, RN-BC, NE-BC, FABC,** is the ANCC Magnet Recognition Program® director for Summa Akron City and St. Thomas Hospitals in Akron, Ohio. She has held a variety of nursing professional development positions, including educator, coordinator, and director, for the past 36 years. Brunt has presented on a variety of topics both locally and nationally and has published 42 articles, five chapters in books, and six books, in addition to an online continuing education module. She served as a section editor for all four editions of *The Core Curriculum for Nursing Professional Development*, published by the National Nursing Staff Development Organization (now known as the Association for Nursing Professional Development).

Brunt holds a master's degree in community health education from Kent State University and a master's in nursing from the University of Dundee in Scotland. Her research has focused on competencies. Brunt maintains certification in nursing professional development and as a nurse executive. She completed a two-year leadership fellowship through The Advisory Board. She has been active in numerous professional associations and has received awards for excellence in writing, nursing research, leadership, and nursing professional development. She was a 2013 nursing excellence regional winner for advancing and leading the profession category through Heartland/ Midwest Nurse.com.

## About the Contributing Author

**Julia W. Aucoin, DNS, RN-BC, CNE,** is certified in Nursing Professional Development and Academic Education and has worked on the certification teams with associated competencies for both specialty practices. She has served as a professor in nursing education and as the CE Consultant for the North Carolina Nurses Association. Dr. Aucoin is a frequent presenter at the Association for Nursing Professional Development and National League for Nursing's Annual Conventions. She is co-editor of *Conversations in Nursing Professional Development*, published by NNSDO.

# Acknowledgments

This book was made possible through the support and assistance of many individuals, and although I cannot recognize everyone who assisted with this endeavor, there are some special people I would like to acknowledge.

First and foremost, I would like to thank the nursing professional development (NPD) specialists throughout the United States who participated in the research studies that led to the development of the competency assessment tool. I asked for feedback and suggestions on the competencies and performance criteria and received a wealth of information from the respondents. This helped me refine and clarify the competencies and performance expectations. When I went back to members of the National Nursing Staff Development Organization (NNSDO), now known as the Association for Nursing Professional Development (ANPD) and asked for feedback on how the competencies fit into Benner's framework, they responded with valuable feedback.

Julia Aucoin is a dear friend and colleague. She provided support, assistance, and encouragement throughout all my research studies. In addition to suggesting I validate the results with academic educators, she helped gather data from a pilot group to gain additional feedback on how the performance criteria fit into Benner's novice-to-expert continuum, prior to the latest research study.

Dr. Liz Rogerson from the University of Dundee in Scotland helped me enhance my critical thinking skills and become a more reflective practitioner. As my dissertation advisor, she provided ongoing feedback in all the stages of this project to help make sense of all the data I had collected.

I would like to thank Summa Health System and particularly Lanie Ward for her ongoing support of my professional endeavors. Summa Health System Foundation and the Department of Patient Care Services provided financial support for the pilot study through the Clinical Ladder program. The Nursing Research Division also provided data analysis assistance throughout all the phases of the research. In addition, I would like to recognize the financial assistance from NNSDO for research grants for four of the phases of the initial study, the Delta Omega Chapter of Sigma Theta Tau for partial support of one phase of the study, and the Ohio Nurses Foundation for financial support for one phase of the study. The latest research was funded through grants from NNSDO and the Delta Omega Chapter of Sigma Theta Tau.

Last, but certainly not least, I want to acknowledge my daughters Rhonda Beasley and Becky Brunt, as well as my mother Betty Johnson. They are an important part of my life and who I am, and I am very lucky to have such wonderful family members who always are there to support and encourage me.

# About This Book

This book is based on the work *Competencies for Staff Educators: Tools to Evaluate and Enhance Nursing Professional Development*, written by Barbara Brunt in 2007.

The work has been updated to reflect the revised *Nursing Professional Development: Scope and Standards of Practice* and includes information on new competencies and performance criteria, as well as a classification of the competencies into Benner's novice-to-expert framework.

All the book's resources are available to download and customize for your practice, including the full listing of competencies.

To access the resources, please visit:

*www.hcpro.com/downloads/12244*.

## Continuing Education

### Nursing contact hours

HCPro is accredited as a provider of continuing nursing education by the American Nurses Credentialing Center's Commission on Accreditation.

This educational activity for 2.7 nursing contact hours is provided by HCPro.

Nursing contact hours for this activity are valid from July 2014 until July 2016.

For complete information about credits available and instructions on how to take the continuing education exam, please visit the downloads page and see the *Nursing Education Instructional Guide* found at *www.hcpro.com/downloads/12244*.

## Disclosure statement

The planners, presenters/authors, and contributors of this CNE activity have disclosed no relevant financial relationships with any commercial companies pertaining to this activity.

## Learning objectives

After reading this book, the participant should be able to:

- Discuss the evolvement of nursing professional development competencies

- Describe the use of Benner's novice-to-expert theory as applied to nursing professional development competencies

- Recognize the role of ANA and NNSDO's *Nursing Professional Development: Scope and Standards of Practice in* creating nursing professional development competencies

- Apply the nursing professional development competencies in professional practice

# List of Figures

Figure 1.1: Comparison of Competency-Based Education (CBE) and Traditional Education ........................6

Figure 1.2: Advantages of Evidence-Based Practice..................................................................................8

Figure 1.3: Core Competencies of Nurse Educators ........................................................................11

Figure 2.1: Overview of the Research Study .....................................................................................14

Figure 3.1: Additional Competencies and Performance Criteria ......................................................20

Figure 4.1: Skill Expectations in Benner's Novice-to-Expert Continuum ........................................34

Figure 4.2: Implications for Teaching Strategies Based on the Five Stages of Skill Acquisition..................37

Figure 5.1: Nursing Professional Development Specialist Practice Model ........................................43

Figure 6.1: Competency Validation Partnership................................................................................50

Figure 6.2: Characteristics of Competency Checklists .....................................................................51

Figure 6.3: Sample Educational Case Study......................................................................................52

Figure 8.1: Advantages and Disadvantages of Nursing Professional Development Structures ..................63

Exhibit 8.1: Nursing Professional Development Job Description .....................................................65

Exhibit 8.2: Director, Nursing Research and Professional Development Job Description ..........................68

Exhibit 8.3: System Director Employee Development Job Description..............................................73

Figure 9.1: Example of an Orientation Program Based on Selected Roles........................................80

Exhibit 9.1: Sample Orientation Schedule for New Medical/Surgical Educator .............................83

Exhibit 10.1: Sample Competency Checklist.....................................................................................90

Exhibit 10.2: Sample Equipment-Related Competency ....................................................................91

Figure 11.1: Professional Values to Consider ...................................................................................96

Figure 12.1: Barriers to Cultural Competence ................................................................................103

Figure 13.1: Best Method of Education to Use With Various Generations......................................111

# Introduction

Although the focus on competence in nursing practice is a worldwide phenomenon and there is a lot of literature on educational methods to achieve competence, there is limited literature on nursing professional development (NPD) competencies or effective methods to measure the achievement of competencies by NPD specialists.

This book, which will add to the body of evidence-based staff development literature, is appropriate for NPD or patient educators in any setting. Since many of the educational competencies are similar regardless of practice setting, this may also be helpful as a resource for educators in other settings, such as academia or consultants.

Individuals can take the competencies in this book and immediately incorporate them into their practice. The book focuses on how to use this information in a variety of ways, such as by creating an orientation for a new staff development specialist, completing a self-assessment, creating criterion-based job descriptions, providing an orientation for new educators, or incorporating them as part of a performance development plan. This will provide a consistent, objective, validated tool to assist NPD educators in measuring their competence. With today's emphasis on cost-containment and accountability, it is critical that educators demonstrate their competence.

This book will provide specific performance criteria to evaluate a wide range of professional NPD educator competencies. The author consolidated information from a series of research studies designed to identify and validate specific criteria that determine whether NPD educators were meeting various competencies and also put in a framework consistent with the latest edition of *Nursing Professional Development: Scope and Standards of Practice* (American Nurses Association and National Nursing Staff Development Organization, 2010).

The book is divided into three sections. The first section provides an overview of the competency movement and describes how the educational competencies and performance criteria in this book were developed, incorporating the latest research on Benner's novice-to-expert framework. It has two new chapters, one detailing the additional competencies based on the revised standards and a chapter on Benner's theory. The framework for the competencies was revised to incorporate Benner's framework. The chapter on methods that can be used to validate competence was updated.

The second section provides examples of how the competencies can be used and applied in the practice setting in a variety of roles. Specific areas include self-assessment, criterion-based position descriptions, orientation, performance appraisals, peer review and professional development plans, professional portfolios, and cultural competence. A new chapter on understanding generational differences was added.

The third section explores other potential uses of the competencies, as well as future trends. A new chapter was included on the educational implications of the Institute of Medicine Report *The Future of Nursing*. The self-assessment tool is included with the rest of the resources on the downloads page, so individuals can easily modify it to meet their individual needs. Please visit *www.hcpro.com/ downloads/12244* to access the downloads.

# Section I

# Competency Assessment and Validation

This section provides an overview of the competency movement and describes how the educational competencies and corresponding performance criteria in this book were developed. There is a new chapter with information on the competencies that were added from the first edition based on the revised *Scope and Standards of Practice* and a new chapter on Benner's novice-to-expert theory. The framework for the competencies is updated to be consistent with the new standards and incorporates results of the latest research on classifying the competencies on Benner's level of expertise. The final chapter in the section outlines methods that can be used to validate competence.

# Chapter 1

# Overview of the Competency Movement

## Learning Objective

**After reading this chapter, the participant should be able to:**

☑ Discuss key components of competence and competency-based education

## Key Concepts

Before beginning a discussion of nursing professional development (NPD) educator competencies, it is important to first discuss the key concepts and definitions. Most of these concepts have been defined in the 2010 edition of the American Nurses Association (ANA) and National Nursing Staff Development Organization (NNSDO) *Nursing Professional Development: Scope and Standards of Practice.*

**Competency:** "An expected level of performance that integrates knowledge, skills, abilities, and judgment" (ANA & NNSDO, 2010, p. 43). Competency focuses on one's actual performance in a situation, which means that competence is required before one can expect to achieve competency (American Board of Nursing Specialties, 2011).

**Core competency:** "A defined fundamental level of knowledge, ability, skill, or expertise that is essential to a particular job" (ANA & NNSDO, 2010, p. 43).

**Professional role competence:** "Performance that meets defined criteria based on the specialty area, context, and model of practice in which an individual nurse in engaged" (ANA & NNSDO, 2010, p. 45).

**Continuing education:** "Those systematic professional learning experiences designed to augment the knowledge, skills, and attitudes of nurses and therefore enrich nurses' contribution to quality healthcare and their pursuit of professional career goals" (ANA & NNSDO, 2010, p. 43).

**Nursing professional development:** "The lifelong process of active participation by nurses to develop and maintain competence, enhance professional nursing practice, and support achievement of their career goals" (ANA & NNSDO, 2010, p. 1).

**Nursing professional development specialist:** "A registered nurse with experience in nursing education who: influences professional role competence and professional growth of nurses in a variety of settings; supports lifelong learning of nurses and other healthcare personnel in an environment that facilitates continuous learning; and fosters an appropriate climate for learning and facilitates the adult learning process" (ANA & NNSDO, 2010, p. 44)

**Performance criteria:** "Statements that define the critical or essential behaviors that represent a particular competency. These outcomes require integration of learning and application of that learning" (Brunt, 2007).

## Why Is Competence Important?

Continuing competence is an issue that affects nurses in all practice settings. Society demands that nurses demonstrate their competence. Increased pressure from multiple healthcare regulatory agencies and the public necessitates comprehensive evaluation of staff competency. In addition, the emphasis on evidence-based practice has created increased scrutiny of clinicians and their preparation.

The issue of continued competence will remain a challenge to the health profession for many years. With ongoing changes in science and technology, the healthcare environment, patient expectations, and regulations, health professionals are challenged to attain and maintain competence throughout their career. However, definitions of competence and strategies to document competence vary, and there is little evidence to support specific, successful methods for validating competence.

## What Is Competence in Nursing?

The focus on competence in nursing is a worldwide phenomenon. Klopper (2013) outlined several themes in her call to action for the Sigma Theta Tau International Honor Society of Nursing. Her overall theme was "Serve locally, transform regionally, and lead globally." This included instituting core competencies and standards for professional nursing practice and developing nurses' competency to assess and use technology and to effectively apply health information. Other themes related to competence include promoting lifelong learning systems for nurses, creating evidence-based nursing models, and developing innovative strategies to educate patients, communities, and nurses.

Most writers agree that competency is about what someone can do. Competency involves both the ability to perform in a given context and the capacity to transfer knowledge and skills to new tasks and situations. Performance criteria outline the steps that must be taken to achieve competency.

Being "competent" in a task or role results from learning outcomes. One of the responsibilities of NPD specialists is to assess the competencies of nursing staff members. NPD specialists have an important role in promoting lifelong learning for nurses and documenting the competence of nursing staff members. These educators build on the education and experiential bases of nurses throughout their professional careers for the ultimate goal of ensuring quality healthcare for the public.

## Competency-Based Education

Competency-based education (CBE) is one approach that NPD specialists use to assess and validate competence. CBE reflects a pragmatic concern for doing, not just knowing how to do. Competency models began to evolve during the 1960s as an approach to education, and today CBE models are a widely applied approach to validating competence. With CBE, the learners' self-direction allows educators to act as facilitators to promote learners' goals. The CBE approach is compatible with adult developmental needs.

Common characteristics of CBE include a learner-centered philosophy, real-life orientation, flexibility, clearly articulated standards, a focus on outcomes, and criterion-reference evaluation methods. CBE emphasizes outcomes in terms of what individuals must know and be able to do and allows flexible pathways for achieving those outcomes. A comparison of CBE and traditional education is provided in Figure 1.1.

Figure 1.1 | Comparison of Competency-Based Education (CBE) and Traditional Education

| Characteristic | CBE programs (learner-centered) | Traditional education (teacher-centered) |
|---|---|---|
| Basis of instruction: | Participant outcomes (competencies) | Specific information to be covered |
| Pace of instruction: | Learner sets own pace in meeting objectives | All proceed at pace determined by instructor |
| How to proceed from task to task: | Master one task before moving to another | Fixed amount of time on each unit/module |
| Focus of instruction: | Specific tasks included in role | Information that may or may not be part of role |
| Method of evaluation: | Criterion referenced | Normative referenced |

*Source: Barbara Brunt. 2004.*

Benefits of a competency-based approach include:

- Encouraging teamwork
- Enhancing skills and knowledge
- Increasing staff retention
- Reducing staff anxiety
- Increasing productivity
- Improving nursing performance
- Ensuring compliance with The Joint Commission (TJC) standard that all members of the staff are competent to fulfill their assigned responsibilities

The American Nurses Credentialing Center's (ANCC) Magnet Recognition Program® (MRP) objectives include promoting quality in a milieu that supports professional nursing practice and promoting positive patient outcomes (ANCC, 2014). The focus on outcomes and involvement of nurses in the decision-making process that is seen in MRP-designated hospitals is consistent with the tenets of the CBE approach for individuals.

## Evidence-Based Practice and Practice-Based Evidence

In the updated model of nursing professional development specialist practice (ANA & NNSDO, 2010), the NPD process is illustrated with a systems model consisting of interrelated inputs, throughputs, outputs, and feedback. Evidence-based practice (EBP) and practice-based evidence (PBE) provide the core of the system throughputs. Competency programs are one of the processes that revolve around EBP and PBE. EBP is the integration of the best research evidence, educational and clinical expertise, and learner values to facilitate decision-making. Complementary to EBP, PBE is a study methodology related more directly to practice effectiveness and improvement that promotes a greater understanding of individual and group differences.

According to Melnyk, Fineout-Overholt, Gallagher-Ford, and Kaplan (2012), EBP is a problem-solving approach to clinical practice that incorporates the best evidence from well-designed studies, patient values, and preferences. This definition not only incorporates research data but also acknowledges patient values. The current focus on EBP has caused increased scrutiny of clinicians and their preparation.

Why is there such an emphasis on EBP? First and foremost, it can lead to better patient outcomes. But it also is a response to pressures for cost containment from payers and healthcare facilities—if better and more efficient treatments are incorporated into practice, then the length of stay should decrease, as will overall costs.

Another reason for the focus on EBP is that consumers today are much more knowledgeable about treatment options. It is not uncommon for patients to go to the Internet to find out more information about a specific disease, test, or treatment. For example, WebMD is one of the most used healthcare sites providing information to consumers. Ultimately, EBP can provide opportunities for nurses to be more effective, and it acknowledges the value of nursing clinical judgment. Advantages of EBP are outlined in Figure 1.2.

Figure 1.2 | Advantages of Evidence-Based Practice

| |
|---|
| Produces better patient outcomes and/or educational outcomes |
| Responds to pressure for cost containment from payers and healthcare facilities, as well as educational administrators |
| Acknowledges increased consumer savvy about treatment and care options and learner savvy about educational strategies |
| Provides opportunities for nursing care and nursing education to be individualized, streamlined, more effective, and dynamic |
| Acknowledges the value of clinical judgment and critical thinking |

Melnyk et al. (2012) described the state of EBP in U.S. nurses. The top five barriers that were identified included:

1. Time
2. Organizational culture
3. Lack of EBP knowledge/education
4. Lack of access to evidence/information
5. Manager/leader resistance

Their study reinforced the tremendous need for nurse executives/leaders to build an organizational culture that supports EBP, implement strategies to enhance nurses' EBP knowledge and skills, and provide environments where EBP can thrive and be sustained.

NPD specialists must provide learning opportunities regarding EBP and facilitate supportive cultures to achieve the Institute of Medicine's goal that 90% of clinical decisions be evidence-based.

Nursing is a complex profession, requiring a good knowledge base and critical thinking skills. The function of nursing education is to produce a competent practitioner, adept in basic knowledge and with the ability to apply critical thinking. Nurse educators play a key role in helping nurses apply EBP concepts to their practice. New approaches to education and practice should be based on research and evidence of best practices. NPD specialists need to conduct research and utilize research findings on the best approaches to education and documentation of competency.

# Competencies for Nursing Professional Development Specialists

We need to ensure we are using evidence of best practice in all aspects of nursing, including education. Historically, there has been little documentation of whether educators are using research-based methods or are competent to do the tasks with which they are entrusted.

There has been some research undertaken and articles published detailing specific competencies for NPD specialists. Brunt (2007) identified research-based competencies of the staff educator role in the first edition of this book. Harper (2013) identified both core competencies and qualifications needed to fulfill the intertwined roles of NPD practice according to the new standards.

Ramsburg and Childress (2012) did an initial investigation of the applicability of the Dreyfus skill acquisition model to the professional development of NPD specialists. The nurse educator role is complex and success requires a commitment to developing a continuum of skill acquisition. The importance of NPD specialist competence can't be overstated; it directly affects the skills and abilities of nurses. A tool was developed and 192 NPD specialists completed it. Participants rated their level of skill acquisition on a 5-point Likert scale. More than 90% of the respondents had a master's degree, post-master's certificate, or doctoral degree, and more than 70% had five years or more of teaching experience.

NPD specialists reported the lowest level of skill acquisition for: a) leading interdisciplinary efforts to address healthcare and education regionally, nationally, and internationally; b) balancing teaching, scholarship, and service; c) participating as a team member in scholarly activities and demonstrating effective proposal writing; d) designing and conducting research; e) disseminating information locally, nationally, and/or internationally to enhance nursing education; and f) advocating for nursing in the political arena. This study provided insight into skill acquisition among NPD specialists, as well as information regarding factors that play a role in knowledge and skill acquisition.

Davis, Stullenbarger, Dearman, and Kelley (2005) reported on the development and validation of competencies to guide the preparation of NPD specialists. They identified 37 competency statements to reflect the knowledge, skills, and abilities that all NPD specialists must demonstrate within the roles of teacher, scholar, and collaborator.

# Difference Between NPD Competencies and Academic Educator Competencies

With the evolution in NPD practice, technology has changed the learning environment and the potential target audiences in both the continuing education and academic education domains. New methods of teaching and learning have developed, requiring changes in the NPD knowledge and expertise to incorporate these into their educational programs. Academic education refers to those courses taken in colleges or universities after the basic nursing education program.

Academic courses may or may not lead to a degree or completion of a certificate program. Continuing education and academic education overlap as nurses select the most effective way to meet their professional development needs and as educators engage in their practice roles. Academic education may be accessed to pursue a specific course of study for a degree or certificate or as individual courses through which to update oneself in a particular area. Continuing education can be part of NPD or part of a formal academic program. Past editions of the scope and standards for NPD practice conceptualized it by three overlapping domains of staff development, continuing education, and academia. However, the updated practice model is based on a systems approach with input, throughputs, and outputs. System inputs include both the learner and the NPD specialist. System throughputs included a number of developmental and educational processes that revolve around EBP and PBE. These processes are orientation, competency program, inservice education, continuing education, career development and role transition, research and scholarship, and academic partnerships. System output and outcomes include learning, change, and professional role competence and growth, leading to protection of the public and provision of quality care. The feedback loops represent the continuing lifelong learning and growth that influences that constantly evolving practice of nursing and NPD (ANA & NNSDO, 2010).

Although some aspects of the educational role are similar across all settings, differences exist in competencies expected in the NPD role and competencies expected of an academic educator in a university setting. The educational process does not change with the setting, so the competencies specific to assessment, planning, implementing, and evaluating educational activities would be the same. Some of the differences are noted below.

Most frequently, academic educators are working with a group of students enrolled in an educational program over a preestablished period of time, usually a semester or quarter. They interact with the same group of students throughout that period and can build on previous sessions as students progress through the curriculum. Frequently, NPD specialists deal with participants in a single session or for very short periods of time. This makes it more difficult to build on information provided in previous sessions.

The National League for Nursing (NLN) identified core competencies of nurse educators. This arose from the Think Tank on Graduate Preparation for the Nurse Educator Role held in December 2001. Members of the Think Tank included faculty and administrators from associate degree, baccalaureate degree, and graduate nursing programs, as well as representatives from staff development and the higher education community. This group generated a list of eight competencies, with several ideas under each competency to further define the scope of each. Following the Think Tank, the Task Group on Nurse Educator Competencies began an extensive search of the literature to determine if the eight competencies were documented in evidence-based literature or if there was a need to modify them. The final list had eight overall competencies, with 66 task statements identified further describing the competencies. The overall competency statements are outlined in Figure 1.3.

**Figure 1.3 | Core Competencies of Nurse Educators**

| |
|---|
| 1. Facilitate learning |
| 2. Facilitate learner development and socialization |
| 3. Use assessment and evaluation strategies |
| 4. Participate in curriculum design and evaluation of program outcomes |
| 5. Function as change agents and leaders |
| 6. Pursue continuous quality improvements in the nurse educator role |
| 7. Engage in scholarship |
| 8. Function within the educational environment |

Source: Adapted from the National League for Nursing. 2005. "Core competencies of nurse educators with task statements." New York: NLN. Retrieved from *www.nln.org/profdev/ corecompetencies.pdf.*

In many instances there are different expectations in the NPD role and academic role with respect to publishing. One of the task statements for the competency on facilitating learner development and socialization deals with dissemination of information through publications. The phrase "publish or perish" is frequently used by academic educators, who must publish to gain tenure. It is an expectation in many universities that faculty publish in peer-reviewed journals in their field. In most NPD specialist roles, this is not a required competency.

One of the task statements under the competency of engaging in scholarship relates to demonstrating skills in proposal writing for initiatives that include, but are not limited to, research, resources acquisition, program development, and policy development. Grant writing is an area that is more commonly seen in academic education. Many NPD specialists do not have any experience with grant writing and may not have the resources to develop expertise in that area. In many arenas, academic educators are expected to write grants and receive funding for their research projects.

The Association for Nursing Professional Development (ANPD), formerly known as NNSDO, is working on a document that will compare and contrast the roles of the NPD and academic educator, which should be available in late 2014.

Coates and Fraser (2014) described the role of the clinical nurse educator, whose primary role is to support the ongoing educational needs of nursing staff, as challenging and extensive. They proposed the creation and strengthening of collaborative networks with academic nurse educators to decrease feelings of isolation, sharing of ideas, reducing duplication of work, ongoing professional development, and mentorship.

This chapter provided an overview of the competency movement, including competency-based education, EBP, and NPD and academic educator competencies.

# References

American Board of Nursing Specialties. (2011, March). Statement on continuing competence for nursing: A resource for action. Retrieved from *http://nursingcertification.org/pdf/CCTF%20Statement%20FINAL%20 032911.pdf*.

American Nurses Association and National Nursing Staff Development Organization. (2010). *Nursing professional development: Scope and standards of practice.* Silver Spring, MD: Nursesbook.org.

American Nurses Credentialing Center. (2014). "ANCC Magnet Recognition Program®." Silver Spring, MD: ANCC. Retrieved from *http://www.nursecredentialing.org/Magnet/ProgramOverview/WhyBecomeMagnet/Value-of-Magnet*.

Brunt, B.A. (2007). *Competencies for staff educators: Tools to evaluate and enhance nursing professional development.* Danvers, MA: HCPro.

Coates, K., & Fraser, K. (2014). A case for collaborative networks for clinical nurse educators. Nurse Education Today, 34, 6–10. *http://dx.doi.org/10.1016/jnedt.2013.04.003*.

Davis, D., Stullenbarger, E., Dearman, C., & Kelley, J.A. (2005). Proposed nurse educator competencies: Development and validation of a model. *Nursing Outlook,* 53, 206–211.

Harper, M. G. (2013). Qualifications of the nursing professional development specialist. In S.L. Bruce (ed.), *Core curriculum for nursing professional development.* (4th ed., pp. 151–179). Chicago, IL: Association for Nursing Professional Development.

Klopper, H.L. (2013). Call to action: Serve locally, transform regionally, lead globally. Retrieved from *http://www.nursingsociety.org/aboutus/board/pages/bio_klopper.aspx*.

Melnyk, B.M., Fineout-Overholt, E., Gallagher-Ford, L., & Kaplan, L. (2012). The state of evidence-based practice in US nurses: Critical implications for nurse leaders and educators. *The Journal of Nursing Administration*, 42(9), 410–417. doi:10.1097/NNA.0b013e3182664e0a.

National League for Nursing (2005). "Core competencies of nurse educators with task statements." New York: NLN. Retrieved from *http://www.nln.org/profdev/corecompetencies.pdf*.

Ramsburg, L., & Childress, R. (2012). An initial investigation of the applicability of the Dreyfus skill acquisition model to the professional development of educators. *Nursing Education Perspective,* 13, 312–316.

# Chapter 2

# Developing Educator Competencies

| Learning Objective |
| --- |
| **After reading this chapter, the participant should be able to:** |
| ☑ Describe the research process used to develop the competencies and performance criteria |

## Performing a Nursing Professional Development Research Study

The performance criteria for the list of nursing professional development (NPD) competencies, included in the appendix, came from extensive research studies completed in three stages over a four-year period. Figure 2.1 provides an overview of research studies.

Figure 2.1 | Overview of the Research Study

| |
|---|
| Starting point: Advanced practice report (NNSDO 1997) that identified key competencies relevant to advanced practice |
| Development of a self-assessment tool with 116 basic and advanced competencies |
| Completion of a pilot study to validate a method to identify performance criteria for 10 competency statements |
| Nine additional studies completed to identify performance criteria for a total of 109 competency statements |
| Validation of survey results for 25 competencies by a group of academic educators |
| Consolidation and grouping of competencies and performance criteria using ANA standards, Harden's model, and Benner's framework |
| Testing of researcher's "novice-to-expert" categorization with a group of local and national nursing professional development educators. |
| Development of initial Nursing Professional Development Educator Competency Tool, published in 2007 |
| Additional competencies added after new standards were published in 2010 |
| Additional research study conducted asking sample participants to classify all the competencies on Benner's novice-to-expert framework |
| Revised competency tool developed using results of latest research study and Benner's framework. |

## Origins of the Competencies

The first stage built upon a Delphi research study on advanced practice competencies completed by the ANA Council on Continuing Education and Staff Development (CE/SD) and the National Nursing Staff Development Organization (NNSDO) in 1995. The goal of the Delphi technique is to reach consensus on a particular topic. A panel of experts gives individual feedback on a subject, which is then judged by the entire panel. The process is repeated, building on information obtained in each round, until some agreement is obtained. The study identified 63 advanced practice competencies in continuing education and staff development.

The author of this book added basic competencies derived from a review of the literature and 20 years of experience in staff development to create a self-assessment tool with 116 competency statements.

When individuals completing the self-assessment tool had questions about how they would know whether they had achieved a particular competency, the primary investigator (PI) identified the need for specific performance criteria.

## Ongoing Research

In the second stage of the study, the researcher eliminated some redundant competencies from the self-assessment tool and started with 109 competency statements, which were all classified as either objective or subjective. Quantitative research methods were used for the objective statements and qualitative methods were used for the subjective statements.

A pilot study was completed to validate the method used to identify performance criteria, and nine additional phases of stage 2 were completed to identify performance criteria for all 109 competencies (Brunt, 1999). For each phase of this study, feedback was obtained from a random, stratified sample of nurses certified in Nursing Professional Development (NPD), as well as regional groups. A description of the method used for the pilot study and subsequent studies is outlined in the 2002 article "Identifying performance criteria for staff development competencies" in the *Journal for Nurses in Staff Development.*

These studies provided a comprehensive description of NPD competencies with specific performance criteria to determine whether an educator met those competencies. These studies established the validity and reliability of an extensive range of competency statements and accompanying performance criteria that could be used by NPD educators with a range of expertise, from novice to expert.

## Validating the Results

Stage 3 involved validating the results of the national and regional samples with a group of academic educators for 25 selected competencies and performance criteria. Nurse faculty members from a list of educators in National League for Nursing accredited baccalaureate and master's nursing programs throughout the United States were invited to participate in an online survey.

This survey used the same Likert scale as the other phases. A Likert scale is a form of response scale commonly used with questionnaires. When responding to a Likert questionnaire item, respondents specify their level of agreement to a given statement. Results from this group were compared with the national sample of certified nurses and regional sample of NNSDO affiliates, to determine whether there were similarities in the competencies and performance criteria across different settings.

## Refining the Results

The final stage of the initial studies refined the competency statements and performance criteria based on the feedback received in stages 2 and 3. The PI analyzed feedback from respondents to reduce duplication in the competency statements and further clarify performance criteria for the competencies.

The statements were consolidated into 72 competencies. For any competency where there was a significant difference between the national and regional results, a small group of expert SD educators (the executive board of NNSDO) was asked to provide additional feedback. The result was a comprehensive, research-based tool to measure the competence of NPD educators (Brunt, 2005, Brunt, 2007).

The information obtained from this study may be applicable to educators in other disciplines and in other settings throughout the United States and the world. Others could replicate the method used in the research to identify performance criteria for other specialties.

## Additional Research

When the updated *Scope and Standard for Nursing Professional Development* was published (ANA & NNSDO, 2010), the author recognized that there were new competencies identified in the standards and also wanted to classify the competencies based on Benner's novice-to-expert framework (Benner, 1984). Details of the seven new competencies are outlined in Chapter 3.

An additional research study was conducted in 2011 to have participants identify where the competencies fit on Benner's framework, using a survey tool. Individuals were also asked to identify what level each of the new competencies fit, in addition to providing feedback on new performance criteria. A sample of nurses belonging to the NNDSO (now known as the Association for Nursing Professional Development) was asked to classify the competencies by level of expertise and also provide feedback on performance criteria for the new competencies. More than 600 surveys were returned. The primary investigator did a content analysis on the feedback from the participants and those data are included in this edition of the book. Statistical tests were completed to identify a level of expertise for each competency.

In the original edition of the standards, six roles were identified: educator, facilitator, change agent, consultant, teacher, and researcher. While these roles are still elements of NPD practice, they are no longer separate roles— but rather they are intertwined as the complexity of NPD practice increases.

The intertwined elements are educator/facilitator, educator/academic liaison, change agent/team member, researcher/consultant, leader/communicator, and collaborator/advisor/mentor. The tool included in the appendix uses the framework of intertwined elements and lists the competency in each element in order of novice to expert based on feedback from the research study.

This chapter provided an overview of the research studies from which the competencies and performance criteria were developed and validated.

## References

American Nurses Association and National Nursing Staff Development Organization. (2010). *Nursing professional development: Scope and standards of practice.* Silver Spring, MD: Nursesbooks.org.

Benner, P. (1984). *From novice to expert: Excellence and power in clinical nursing practice.* Menlo Park, CA: Addison-Wesley.

Brunt, B.A. (1999). *Competencies of staff development educators: Personal assessment of competency.* Akron, OH: Summa Health System.

Brunt, B.A. (2002). Identifying performance criteria for staff development competencies, *Journal for Nurses in Staff Development, 18*(4), 213–217.

Brunt, B.A. (2005). Identifying performance criteria for staff development competencies. Unpublished master's dissertation. University of Dundee, Scotland.

National Nursing Staff Development Organization. (1997). *Report of the Task Force on Advanced Practice in Nursing Continuing Education and Staff Development.* Pensacola, FL: NNSDO.

Brunt, B.A. (2007). *Competencies for staff educators: Tools to evaluate and enhance nursing professional development.* Danvers, MA: HCPro.

# Chapter 3

# Additional Competencies Based on Revised Standards

## Learning Objective

**After reading this chapter, the participant should be able to:**

☑ Describe key components of the additional competencies

## Additional Competencies

When the new standards (American Nurses Association [ANA] and National Nursing Staff Development Organization [NNSDO], 2010) were published, the author identified additional competencies that were not included in her original work. This chapter will detail information on these seven competencies, which are:

1. Demonstrates proficiency in use of technology

2. Oversees evidence-based practice (EBP) and practice-based evidence (PBE)

3. Assists with excellence initiatives, such as ANCC Magnet Recognition Program® (MRP) and the Malcolm Baldrige National Quality Award (MBNQA)

4. Incorporates transformational leadership principles into practice

5. Promotes career development and role transition

6. Facilitates peer review

7. Demonstrates emotional intelligence

Figure 3.1 lists the competency statements and corresponding performance criteria for these competencies.

Figure 3.1 | Additional Competencies and Performance Criteria

---

Demonstrates proficiency in use of technology
1.  Demonstrates information literacy (recognizes information is needed and has the ability to locate, evaluate, and use needed information effectively)
2.  Participates in efforts to improve information management and communication
3.  Integrates technology-enhanced experiences into educational programs
4.  Safeguards privacy and security of information gained through technology
5.  Uses information applications designed for nursing to enhance evidence-based practice and evaluate outcomes of care
6.  Supports patient safety initiatives using information technology

---

Oversees evidence-based practice (EBP) and practice-based evidence (PBE)
1.  Assists staff to gather evidence through various means (classes, journal clubs, etc.)
2.  Supports staff in evaluating various evidence-based options
3.  Encourages integration of EBP and PBE into practice
4.  Plans, implements, and evaluates activities to foster the development of EBP and PBE
5.  Implements evidence-based approaches in policy development

---

Assists with excellence initiatives, such as ANCC Magnet Recognition Program® activities and Malcolm Baldrige National Quality Award
1.  Compares criteria for excellence initiatives to current state (gap analysis)
2.  Uses information from organization or unit (balanced scorecard, quality indicators) to track progress toward desired goals
3.  Fosters creativity, innovation, and willingness to take risks
4.  Tracks and trends patient care and other outcomes
5.  Support professional development, e.g., certification and additional education

---

Incorporates transformational leadership principles into practice
1.  Creates infrastructure that ensures access to information, resources, and support
2.  Sets clear goals and establishes rewards for success
3.  Encourages autonomy, authority, and accountability
4.  Demonstrates skills in strategic planning, advocacy, influence, and communication
5.  Exhibits transformational leadership behaviors, such as trust, integrity, inspiration, and coaching

---

Promotes career development and role transition
1.  Assists individuals to find opportunities for personal growth and development
2.  Promotes professional empowerment (power and authority)
3.  Mentors or facilitates mentoring opportunities for staff
4.  Coordinates or conducts and evaluates activities to promote career development and role transition
5.  Helps promote succession planning for others and self

Figure 3.1 | Additional Competencies and Performance Criteria (cont.)

Facilitates peer review

1. Facilitates the peer review process by fostering a culture that supports sharing with others
2. Participates in systematic peer review
3. Assists with development of peer review tools, as appropriate
4. Educates staff in process and benefits of peer review
5. Seeks feedback regarding own practice

Demonstrates emotional intelligence

1. Incorporates emotional intelligence principles into education activities
2. Promotes an environment that assists staff to deal with the emotional impact of work-related issues
3. Enhances emotional intelligence through training, counseling, and feedback
4. Demonstrates emotional responsiveness through self-awareness, self-regulation, motivation, empathy, and social skills

# Technology

The nursing professional development (NPD) specialist needs a strong knowledge base in innovative technological options (ANA & NNSDO, 2010). Given the rapid technological advances, information cannot be accessed at a rapid pace via the Internet and mobile devices. Information is constantly changing, and nurses must keep their knowledge up to date. NPD specialists need to demonstrate information literacy, which is recognizing that information is needed and having the ability to locate, evaluate, and use needed information effectively.

Along with all health professions, nursing education often uses online instructional methods, with less emphasis on in-person classroom learning. Limited resources and training time necessitate implementation of the most efficient delivery method, minimizing cost, and maximizing learning and performance. NPD specialists need knowledge of technological advances so that they integrate these into learning activities as appropriate to help the critical thinking skills of learners (Holtschneider, 2013). NPD specialists need to participate in efforts to improve information management and communication.

There are a variety of technologies for learning, including computer-based training, conferencing technology options, Web conferencing and webcasts, electronic presentations, social networking and social learning, and simulation (Holtschneider, 2013). NPD specialists need to integrate technology-enhanced experiences into educational programs.

With the advent of information available through technology, NPD specialists must safeguard the privacy and security of information gained through technology. Considerations for electronic records include the following: "The ethical duty of confidentiality entails keeping information shared during the course of a professional relationship secure and secret from others. This obligation involves making appropriate security arrangements for the storage and transmission of private information, and ensuring that the equipment used for storage and transmission is secure." (Brady-Schluttner, 2013, pp. 461–462)

Clinical information systems, which support workflow and EBP, are growing at a rapid pace. Education and training of staff on these information systems is often facilitated through a train-the-trainer or super-user model. NPD specialists need to use information applications designed for nursing to enhance EBP and evaluate outcomes of care.

Patient safety is a growing concern with the increased attention on the number of medical errors. The Institute of Medicine (IOM) published a seminal work in 2000, *To Err is Human: Building a Safer Health System*. NPD specialists need to support patient safety initiatives using information technology.

The performance criteria for the competency "Demonstrates proficiency in the use of technology" are as follows:

- Demonstrates information literacy (recognizes information is needed and has the ability to locate, evaluate, and use needed information effectively).
- Participates in efforts to improve information management and communication.
- Integrates technology-enhanced experiences into educational programs.
- Safeguards privacy and security of information gained through technology.
- Uses information applications designed for nursing to enhance EBP and evaluate outcomes of care.
- Supports patient safety initiatives using information technology.

# EBP and PBE

EBP and PBE form the core of the nursing professional development model. EBP and PBE combine to contribute to the professional growth of practicing nurses and other learners. These are defined as follows:

**EBP:** the integration of the best research evidence, educational and clinical expertise, and learner values to facilitate decision-making. (ANA & NNSDO, 2010, p. 43)

**PBE:** a study methodology related more directly to practice effectiveness and improvement and that promotes a greater understanding of individual and group differences. (ANA & NNSDO, p. 45)

The NPD specialist is a facilitator and role model for staff on ways to gather evidence. This can be done through a variety of methods, such as classes, journal clubs, literature review, etc. If the educator consistently uses evidence in presentations and when discussing options for care, participants can see the value of using evidence in their care.

There is a lot of information easily accessible through various Internet and print sources, but not all of that information is accurate or beneficial. One of the roles of the NPD specialist is to help staff members evaluate sources of information for credibility. Staff members often struggle with identifying what information is appropriate to put into practice and what information needs further validation.

The NPD specialist plays a crucial role in encouraging and role-modeling the integration of EBP and PBE into practice. Melnyk, Gallagher-Ford, Long, and Fineout-Overholt (2014) conducted a study to develop a set of clear EBP competencies for both practice registered nurses (RN) and advanced practice nurses (APN) that can be used by healthcare institutions. Seven national EBP leaders developed an initial set of competencies through a consensus-building process. Then a Delphi survey was conducted with 80 EBP members across the United States to determine consensus and clarity around the competencies. Two rounds of the Delphi survey demonstrated total consensus by the EPB mentors, resulting in a final set of 13 competencies for practicing RNs and 11 additional competencies for APNs. Incorporation of these competencies into healthcare system expectations, orientations, job descriptions, performance appraisals, and clinical-ladder promotion processes could drive high quality, reliability and consistency of healthcare, as well as reduce costs (Melnyk et al., 2014).

When planning, implementing, and evaluating programs, the NPD specialist needs to plan activities to foster the development of EBP and PBE. One tool that has been used to identify factors affecting the implementation of EBP is the Evidence-Based Practice Questionnaire (EBPQ). Upton, Upton, and Scurlock-Evans (2014) did a methodological and narrative literature review of the reach, transferability, and impact of this tool. Technology plays a key role in EBP, such as when searching for information online. One study reported by Upton et al (2014) found confidence using computers was a facilitator of EBP implementation. Targeted skills workshops could be developed to address the needs of the workforce to help overcome barriers related to technology. However, the educator needs to assess the organizational culture and staff learning needs prior to the development of educational interventions to ensure effectiveness.

Another area to implement evidence-based approaches is in the development and review of policies and procedures. The NPD specialist can implement or facilitate implementation of current evidence when reviewing or updating policies. Many organizations now include the references used somewhere within the policy to show others that it was developed or updated with current references.

The performance criteria for the competency "Oversees EBP and PBE" are:

- Assists staff to gather evidence through various means (e.g., classes, journal clubs)

- Supports staff in evaluating various evidence-based options

- Encourages integration of EBP and PBE into practice

- Plans, implements, and evaluates activities to foster the development of EBP and PBE

- Implements evidence-based approaches in policy development

## Excellence Initiatives

With the focus on quality and excellence in healthcare, the NPD specialist often is involved in assisting with the application process. Two well-known initiatives are the MRP and the MBNQA.

The MRP recognizes healthcare organizations for quality patient care, nursing excellence, and innovations in professional nursing practice. Consumers rely on MRP designation as the ultimate credential for high-quality nursing. Developed by the American Nurses Credentialing Center (ANCC), MRP is the leading source of successful nursing practices and strategy worldwide. The MRP requires organizations to develop, disseminate, and enculturate evidence-based criteria that result in a positive work environment for nurses. (ANCC, 2013)

The MBNQA is presented annually by the president of the United States to organizations that demonstrate quality and performance excellence. These awards may be given annually in each of six categories, one of which is healthcare. Organizations that apply for the MBNQA are judged by an independent board of examiners. Recipients are selected based on achievement and improvement in seven areas: leadership; strategic planning; customer and market focus; measurement, analysis, and knowledge management; human resource focus; process management; and business/organizational performance results (Malcolm Baldrige, 2014).

One of the first steps in applying for one of these excellence awards is comparing the criteria for the award to the current state of the organization, which is referred to as a gap analysis. The NPD specialist often assists with this process. Identifying areas for improvement can help focus educational efforts and other activities to put processes into place to meet the criteria.

Because both of these initiatives focus on quality, the NPD specialist may be used to look at the organization's current quality metrics to track progress toward goals. These might be included on the unit or organization's balanced scorecard or in the quality indicator reporting format for the institution. The goal would be the desired state, and the metric indicates where the unit or organization is in meeting that indicator.

One of the hallmarks of MRP status is innovation. Nurses are encouraged and rewarded for innovations in practice (ANCC 2014). The ability to foster creativity and innovation and creating an environment where the individual is comfortable taking risks are critical components in an MRP organization. The NPD specialist can facilitate such an environment and reward individuals for taking risks.

Performance results and quality patient care are criteria for both awards. The NPD specialist can help track and trend patient care and other outcomes. Whether it is nursing-sensitive indicators, patient satisfaction, or overall performance, everyone needs to be aware of the goals/benchmarks and where the organization is in relation to those items.

Having a competent workforce contributes to successful outcomes. The NPD specialist can support professional development of the staff. That can be achieved through certification or additional formal or continuing education. The NPD specialist may facilitate review courses for certification, and the organization may support that with monetary assistance for the certification preparation or the certification exam. Many organizations provide continuing education for their nurses, and many support academic education through tuition assistance programs.

The performance criteria for the competency "Assists with excellence initiatives, such as MRP and MBNQA" are:

- Compares criteria for excellence initiative to current state (gap analysis)
- Uses information from organization or unit (balanced scorecard, quality indicators) to track progress toward desired goals
- Fosters creativity, innovation, and willingness to take risks
- Tracks and trends patient care and other outcomes
- Supports professional development (e.g., certification and additional education)

# Transformational Leadership

Transformational leadership is one of the components of the MRP model. The transformational leader must lead people where they need to meet the demands of the future. This requires vision, influence, clinical knowledge, and a strong expertise relating to professional nursing practice. It also acknowledges that transformation may create turbulence and involve atypical approaches to solutions. The organization's senior leadership team creates the vision for the future and the systems and environment necessary to achieve that vision. They must enlighten the organization as to why change is necessary and communicate each department's part in achieving that change. They must listen, challenge, influence, and affirm as the organization makes its way into the future. (ANCC, 2013)

One of the key components of transformational leadership is having an infrastructure that ensures access to information, resources, and support, which can lead to positive patient outcomes. This was validated in a systematic review done by Wong, Cummings, and Durcharme (2013). They analyzed

20 research studies conducted between 2003 and 2013 and found that current evidence suggests relationships between position relational leadership styles and higher patient satisfaction and lower patient mortality, medication errors, restraint use, and hospital-acquired infections.

A transformational leader sets clear goals and establishes rewards for success. Ensuring nurse autonomy, authority, and accountability are hallmarks of a transformational leader. Lievens and Vlerick (2013) identified how a transformational leadership style can enhance nurses' compliance with and participation in safety. Furthermore, transformational leaders are able to influence the perceptions that their nurses have about the kind and amount of knowledge in their job, which can lead to an increase in both dimensions of nurses' safety performance.

Skills in strategic planning, advocacy, influence, and communication are essential for a trans-formational leader. Broome (2013) conducted a study on self-reported leadership styles of deans of baccalaureate and higher degree nursing programs. Behaviors that the deans reported they frequently, if not always, engaged in were:

- I seek differing perspectives when solving problems
- I talk optimistically about the future
- I talk enthusiastically about what needs to be accomplished
- I specify the importance of having a strong sense of purpose
- I treat others as individuals rather than just part of a group
- I go beyond self-interest for the good of the group
- I articulate a compelling vision for the future
- I help others to develop their strengths
- I express satisfaction when others meet expectations
- I am effective in representing others to higher authority
- I lead a group that is effective

Behaviors seen in transformational leaders include trust, integrity, inspiration, and coaching.

The performance criteria for the competency "Incorporate transformational leadership principles into practice" are:

- Creates infrastructure that ensures access to information, resources, and support
- Sets clear goals and establishes rewards for success
- Encourages nurse autonomy, authority, and accountability
- Demonstrates skills in strategic planning, advocacy, influence, and communication
- Exhibits transformational leadership behaviors, such as trust, integrity, inspiration, and coaching

# Career Development and Role Transition

Career development is one of the core competencies identified in the revised standards. It involves identification and development of strategies that meet the career goals, tasks, and challenges in different stages throughout a nurse's career (ANA & NNSDO, 2010). This can involve career coaching, creating/supporting clinical advancement models, academic education coaching, assisting in role transition, or planning for succession (Setter, 2013).

One of the key components of this process is to help individuals find opportunities for personal growth and development for whatever career development option they are seeking. This can be done through encouraging, teaching, sponsoring, and guiding nurses through significant points in their career.

Career coaching requires effective communication skills, trust, and mutual respect and fosters creative thinking and high expectations. The NPD specialist needs to promote personal empowerment (power and authority) in the individual, so he or she feels prepared for the next step to meet the desired goal.

Mentoring individuals or facilitating mentoring opportunities for staff can help promote career development and role transition. This provides a mechanism for professional growth and development in the individual and lets him or her experience opportunities that might not have been available without a mentor.

There are many activities that can be coordinated or conducted to promote career development and role transition. College fairs, programs on various topics, information on clinical advancement opportunities, and/or shadowing experiences can help individuals identify whether something will meet their career goals.

Another aspect of career development is succession planning. The NPD specialist can help identify potential talent, facilitate training and development opportunities, design comprehensive training and leadership classes, recommend mentors/coaches, create role-related education, and support practical experiences (Setter, 2013).

Performance criteria for the competency "Promotes career development and role transition" are:

- Assists individuals to find opportunities for personal growth and development
- Promotes professional empowerment (power and authority)
- Mentors or facilitates mentoring opportunities for staff
- Coordinates or conducts and evaluates activities to promote career development and role transition
- Helps promote succession planning for others and self

# Peer Review

Peer review is a collegial, systematic, and periodic process by which RNs are held accountable for practice and that fosters the refinement of one's knowledge, skills, and decision-making at all levels and in all areas of practice. (ANA & NNSDO, 2010)

Successful peer review requires a culture that welcomes and values feedback from others. The NPD specialist can help foster a continuous learning culture to facilitate the peer review process. A peer is an individual of the same rank or standing according to the established standards of practice.

The goal of peer review is to improve quality and safety and provide constructive feedback. The NPD specialist can help promote accountability and critical thinking in the peer review process by assisting to identify measurable objectives of performance to guide peers in evaluating each nurse by providing focused, pertinent feedback. Davis, Kenny, Doyle, McCarroll, and von Gruenigen (2013) described a successful peer review program to improve the late deceleration recognition and intervention on one labor and delivery unit. Monthly chart audits met the goal of 75% reviewer agreement after the fourth month of implementation and have been maintained since then. Institutional support, a dedicated review team, and education contributed to success.

NPD specialists should also participate in systematic peer review on a regular basis to enhance their practice. Participating in systematic peer review and seeking feedback regarding one's own practice from learners, professional partners, peers, and supervisors or other administrators as appropriate are two of the measurement criteria in the professional practice evaluation standard (ANA & NNSDO, 2010). Seeking feedback from colleagues and others can be helpful to improve performance.

Tools are helpful in providing consistent evaluation of peers. The NPD specialist may assist with the development of peer review tools. A well-defined peer review process and tool, utilized in conjunction with a nurse's annual performance evaluation, is one way to infuse meaningful peer input into a performance appraisal. This system allowed nurses to provide insight into one another's strengths and opportunities for growth (Ray & Meyer, 2014).

Performance criteria for the competency "Facilitates peer review" are:
- Facilitates the peer review process by fostering a culture that supports sharing with others
- Participates in systematic peer review
- Assists with development of peer review tools, as appropriate
- Educates staff in process and benefits of peer review
- Seeks feedback regarding own practice

# Emotional Intelligence

Emotional intelligence (EI) is defined as the ability to distinguish feeling, to motivate ourselves, and to manage emotions in ourselves and in our relationships. Five dimensions of EI are self-knowledge, self-management and self-regulation, motivation, social awareness, and relationship management (Powell & Kusama-Powell, 2010).

The NPD specialist should demonstrate emotional responsiveness through self-awareness, self-regulation, motivation, empathy, and social skills. Powell and Kusama-Powell (2010) pointed out that before educators can be emotionally sensitive to learners, they need to be emotionally sensitive to themselves.

When the NPD specialist is planning or presenting educational activities, he or she should incorporate EI principles into that education. Emotionally intelligent teachers understand that learning is a voluntary act on the part of the learner. Knowing this, the NPD specialist can create conditions for learning.

The NPD specialist can enhance EI in others through training, counseling, motivation, and feedback. Many individuals are not aware of the concepts of EI, and the NPD specialist can provide educational activities on this topic and counsel individuals with low EI on methods to increase emotional responsiveness.

Working in healthcare can be very emotionally draining. Creating an environment that assists staff to deal with the emotional impact of work-related issues is an important part of the NPD role. Littlejohn (2012) noted that recent research on emotional intelligence suggests that it is possible to improve the emotional competence of adults. Individuals with high EI are able to deal with environmental demands and workplace stress.

The performance criteria for the competency "Demonstrates EI" are:

- Incorporates EI principles into educational activities
- Promotes an environment that assists staff to deal with the emotional impact of work-related issues
- Enhances EI through training, counseling, motivation, and feedback
- Demonstrates emotional responsiveness through self-awareness, self-regulation, motivation, empathy, and social skills

This chapter provided some background on the seven new competencies and corresponding performance criteria that were added since the previous edition of this book.

# References

American Nurses Credentialing Center. (2013). *2014 Magnet Application Manual.* Silver Spring, MD: American Nurses Credentialing Center.

American Nurses Association and National Nursing Staff Development Organization. (2010). *Nursing professional development: Scope and standards of practice.* Silver Spring, MD: Nursesbooks.org.

Brady-Schluttner, K. (2013). Record Keeping. In S.L. Bruce (ed.), *Core curriculum for nursing professional development.* (4th ed., pp. 453–469). Chicago, IL: Association for Nursing Professional Development.

Broome, M.E. (2013). Self-reported leadership styles of deans of baccalaureate and higher degree nursing programs in the United States. *Journal of Professional Nursing,* 29(6), 323–329. *http://dx.doi.org/10.1016/j.profnurs.2013.09.001.*

Davis, J.,Kenny, T.H., Doyle, J.L., McCarroll, M., & von Gruenigen, V.E. (2013). Nursing peer review of late deceleration recognition and intervention to improve patient safety. *Journal of Obstetric, Gynecologic, and Neonatal Nursing,* 42(2), 215–224. doi: 10.1111/1552-6909.12023.

Holtschneider, M.E. (2013). Technology and nursing professional development. In S.L. Bruce (ed.), *Core curriculum for nursing professional development.* (4th ed., pp. 527–545). Chicago, IL: Association for Nursing Professional Development.

Institute of Medicine (2000). *To Err Is Human.* Washington, DC: National Academies Press.

Lievens, I., & Vlerick, P. (2103). Transformational leadership and safety performance among nurses: The mediating role of knowledge-related job characteristics. *Journal of Advanced Nursing,* 70(3), 651–661. doi 10.1111/jan.12229.

Littlejohn, P. (2012). The missing link: Using emotional intelligence to reduce workplace stress and workplace violence in out nursing and other health care professions. *Journal of Professional Nursing,* 28, 360–368. Retrieved from *http://dx.doi.org/10.1016/j.profnurs.2012.05.006.*

Magnet® Recognition Program Overview. (2014). Retrieved from *http://www.nursecredentialing.org/Magnet/ProgramOverview.aspx.*

Melnyk, B.M., Gallagher-Ford, L., Long, L.E., & Fineout-Overholt, E. (2014). The establishment of evidence-based practice competencies for practicing registered nurses and advanced practice nurses in real-world clinical settings: Proficiencies to improve healthcare quality, reliability, patient outcomes, and costs. *Worldviews on Evidence-Based Nursing,* 11(1), 5-15. doi: 10.1111/wvn12021.

Malcolm Baldrige National Quality Award (MBNQA) Overview (2014). Retrieved from *http://asq.org/learn-about-quality/malcolm-baldrige-award/overview/overview.html.*

Powell, W., & Kusuma-Powell, O. (2010). *Becoming an emotionally intelligent teacher.* Thousand Oaks, CA: Corwin.

Ray, K., & Meyer, S. (2014). Moving toward a more objective peer review process. *Nursing Management,* 45(1), 52–54. Doi:10.1097/01.NUMA000043778.30595.be.

Setter, R. (2013). Career development and role transition. In S.L. Bruce (ed.), *Core curriculum for nursing professional development* (4th ed., pp. 515–525). Chicago, IL: Association for Nursing Professional Development.

Upton, D., Upton, P., & Scurlock-Evans, L. (2014). The reach, transferability, and impact of the evidence-based practice questionnaire: A methodological and narrative literature review. *Worldviews on Evidence-Based Nursing,* 11(1), 46-54, 1–9. doi: 10.1111/wvn.12019.

Wong, C.A., Cummings, G.C., & Ducharme, L. (2013). The relationship between nursing leadership and patient outcomes: A systematic review update. *Journal of Nursing Management,* 21, 709–724. doi: 10.1111/jonm.12116.

# Chapter 4

# Benner's Novice-to-Expert Continuum

| Learning Objectives |
| --- |
| **After reading this chapter, the participant should be able to:** |
| ☑  Describe the components of Benner's novice-to-expert theory |
| ☑  Identify applications of Benner's theory in practice |

Benner's seminal work (1984) differentiated practical and theoretical knowledge and built on the Dreyfus model of skill acquisition to develop her novice-to-expert theory.

Key concepts in her theory are defined below (George, 2011, p. 581, 582, 588, 589)

**Assumptions, expectations, and sets:** Beliefs generated from past experience that orient and influence the nurse's perception of the present situation. Sets are subtle and may not be completely explicit. These sets predispose the nurse to act in certain ways when involved in certain situations.

**Background meaning:** Part of context and is the culturally acquired set of meanings the person accumulates from birth. Background meaning is how the world is understood to "be" and influences one's perception of the factual world.

**Caring:** An essential skill of nurses and is "a basic way of being in the world."

**Clinical judgment:** Recognizing salient, or important, aspects of the situation as they unfold and acting appropriately on that knowledge.

**Clinical reasoning:** A process of understanding a particular patient's condition at a particular time based on the changes or transitions observed for that patient.

**Common meanings:** Nurses form common meanings with other nurses in their perspective on health and illness–related issues commonly encountered. These meanings form a tradition that is used to compare specific patient situations and theory and further define common meaning.

**Domains of practice:** Thematic grouping of clinical competencies identified in the narrative account of nurses.

**Graded qualitative distinctions:** The subtle context-dependent physiologic changes experienced by the patient that are recognizable to the expert nurse based on direct patient observation.

**Maxims:** Instructions experts use to pass on explanations of their actions to others.

**Paradigm cases and personal knowledge:** Past situations that stand out in the nurse's memory that allow for rapid perceptual grasp of the situation.

**Unplanned practices:** Practices that have been given to nurses by default. Many unplanned practices are the result of taking on more roles that were once the domain of other healthcare professionals.

Benner identified six areas of practical knowledge, which were: 1) graded qualitative distinctions; 2) common meanings; 3) assumptions, expectations, and sets; 4) paradigm cases and personal knowledge; 5) maxims; and 6) unplanned practices. Adequate description of practical knowledge is essential to the development and extension of nursing theory.

## Dreyfus Model of Skill Acquisition

Stuart Dreyfus, a mathematician and system analyst, and Hubert Dreyfus, a philosopher, developed a model of skill acquisition based upon the study of chess players and airplane pilots. They posited that in the acquisition and development of a skill a student passes through five levels of proficiency: novice, advanced beginner, competent, proficient, and expert. These different levels reflect changes in three general aspects of skilled performance. First is a movement from reliance on abstract principles to the use of past concrete experience as paradigms. Second is a change in the learner's perception of the demand situations, in which the situation is seen less and less as a compilation of equally relevant bits and more and more as a complete whole in which only certain parts are relevant. Third is a passage from detached observer to involved performer (Benner, 1984).

Benner applied the Dreyfus model to nursing through individual and group paired interviews with beginning nurses and nurses recognized for their expertise. Through analysis of that data, she described the performance characteristics at each level of development and identified the teaching/ learning needs of each level. It should be noted that this is a situational model—any nurses entering an area where they have no experience would be considered a novice, regardless of the number of years of experience.

## Stage 1: Novice

Beginners have had no experience of the situations in which they are expected to perform. They rely on context-free rules for drawing conclusions, based on recognizable objective features of the situation. Their behavior is limited and inflexible, as learned rules cannot differentiate relevant versus nonrelevant aspects of the situation. To give them time to gain the experience necessary for skill development, the preceptor or NPD specialist can give them the features of the task that can be recognized without situational experience, focusing on rules to guide performance.

## Stage 2: Advanced beginner

Advanced beginners are nurses who can demonstrate marginally acceptable performance, who have coped with enough real situations to note the recurring meaningful situational components, or aspects, of a situation. They begin to notice some of the situational elements in addition to the objective elements. The NPD specialist or preceptor can provide guidelines for recognizing aspects. Advanced beginners need support and help in setting priorities, since they operate on general guidelines and are only beginning to perceive recurrent meaningful patterns in their clinical practice.

## Stage 3: Competent

Competence, typified by the nurse who has been on the job in the same or similar situations two to three years, develops when the nurse begins to see his or her actions in terms of long-range goals or plans through conscious awareness. Clinical knowledge becomes integrated with theoretical knowledge to allow the nurse to begin to see the big picture. The competent nurse lacks the speed and flexibility of the proficient nurse but does have a feeling of mastery and the ability to cope with and manage the many contingencies of clinical nursing. Nurses at this stage can benefit from decision-making games and simulations that give them practice in planning and coordinating multiple, complex patient care demands.

## Stage 4: Proficient

The proficient nurse perceives situations as a whole rather than in terms of aspects, and performance is guided by maxims. Perceptions are not thought out but present themselves based on experience and recent events. These nurses understand a situation as a whole because they perceive its meaning in terms of long-term goals. The big picture now guides the nurse's care. Proficient nurses are best taught inductively, by beginning with a clinical situation and having the performer supply his or her ways of understanding the situation.

## Stage 5: Expert

The expert nurse no longer relies on rules or maxims to connect an understanding of the situation to an appropriate action but has an intuitive grasp of each situation. This intuition leads to a focus on actions rather than problems. Capturing descriptions of expert performance is difficult, because the expert operates from a deep understanding of the total situation and has difficulty describing the thinking process to reach a decision. Systematic documentation of expert clinical performance is a first step in clinical knowledge development, and expert clinicians can benefit from systematically recording and describing critical incidences from their practice that illustrate expertise.

See Figure 4.1.

Figure 4.1 | Skill Expectations in Benner's Novice-to-Expert Continuum

| Novice | No experience or background with the skill; needs structure and specific guidelines for performance |
|---|---|
| Advanced beginner | Some experience with application of knowledge and skill, but still needs considerable guidance; has difficulty setting priorities; lacks flexibility |
| Competent | Basic comfort level with application of knowledge and skill; conscious deliberate problem solving; sets priorities; sees actions in terms of long-range goals/performance |
| Proficient | Comfortable enough with application of knowledge and skills to adjust priorities based on anticipated response; perceives situation as a whole; performance is guided by subtle nuances |
| Expert | Extensive background and mastery of application of knowledge and skill; intuitive grasp of the situation; able to adjust spontaneously as needed |

Benner's work over several decades has focused on the understanding of perception acuity, clinical judgment, skilled know-how, ethical comportment, and ongoing experiential learning. Ethical comportment relates to the belief that good conduct is a product of an individual relationship with the patient that involves engagement in a situation combined with a sense of membership in a profession. Professional conduct is socially embedded, lived, and embodied in the practice, ways of being, and responses to clinical situations that promote patient well-being, where clinical and ethical judgments are inseparable (Masters, 2012).

Benner identified 31 competencies that were inductively put into seven domains, which are:

1. The helping role
2. The teaching-coaching function
3. The diagnostic and patient-monitoring function
4. Effective management of rapidly changing situations
5. Administering and monitoring therapeutic interventions and regimens
6. Monitoring and ensuring the quality of healthcare practices
7. Organizational work-role competencies (Masters, 2012)

Benner's theory has been widely used throughout the world to describe the progression of clinical expertise. However, Gobet and Chassy (2008) felt that Benner's theory was too simple to account for the complex pattern of phenomena that recent research on expert intuition has uncovered, and they proposed an alternative theory of expert intuition in nursing, known as TempT. A key assumption of TempT is that experts are hampered by the same cognitive limit as novices. For example, attention can be focused on only one thing at a time, and visual short-term memory is limited to just four items. The difference in novices and experts are the number of perceptual patterns, known as chunks. Some patterns that recur often in the environment may lead to the construction not only of chunks, but also of more complex data structures known as templates. Templates possess both a core, which encodes stable information, and slots, which encode variable information. Chunks and templates can be associated with long-term memory information. Expertise is made possible by a large number of chunks and templates that are linked to possible actions.

## Educating Nurses

Benner, Sutphen, Leonard, and Day (2010) conducted a study and proposed a radical transformation in nursing education. The author's analysis revealed three major findings. Most important, U.S. nursing programs were found to be pedagogically strong and effective in forming professional identity and ethical comportment. Second, the clinical practice working directly with real patients, inherent in nursing education, provides a powerful learning experience for students, especially when faculty integrate classroom and clinical teaching. With this second finding, the authors concluded that nursing faculty observed frequently have a disconnect between the classroom lecture, where student passively receive information, and the application of clinical knowledge and judgment in the clinical setting. The authors also concluded that nursing programs are not effective for teaching nursing sciences, natural or social sciences, technology, or the humanities.

Benner and her colleagues included three paradigm cases of excellent teaching and then had a fourth section detailing the kind of teaching and learning that today's profession demands. Because nursing practice demands depth and breadth of knowledge in many areas, the problem of asking students to learn a great deal in a brief period must be resolved. They suggested the following structural changes in nursing education:

- Requiring the baccalaureate degree as the entry into practice
- Introducing nursing courses in the first year of the baccalaureate program
- Increasing second degree baccalaureate and master's programs
- Improving students' efficient progress through Associate Nursing degree programs to baccalaureate and master's programs
- Requiring a postgraduate year of internship in a clinical setting

They suggested that teachers change their assumptions about teaching and their approach to fostering learning in four ways:

1. Shift from a focus on covering decontextualized knowledge to an emphasis on teaching for a sense of salience, situated cognition, and action in particular situations.

2. Shift from a sharp separation from clinical and classroom teaching to integration of classroom and clinical teaching.

3. Shift from an emphasis on critical thinking to an emphasis on clinical reasoning and multiple ways of thinking that include critical thinking.

4. Shift from an emphasis on socialization and role taking to an emphasis on formation. Formation refers to the method by which a person is prepared for a particular task or is made capable of functioning in a particular role.

These concepts and ideas have implications for NPD specialist practice.

## Applications of Benner's Theory

There have been many studies completed using Benner's theory. The author chose three studies to show applications for nurses, managers, and educators.

Dole, Drews, Dimitt, Hildebrandt, Hittle, and Tielsch-Goddard (2013) described the development of an advanced practice evaluation tool. Using Benner's theory, a performance excellence and accountability tool (PEAC Tool©) was designed to measure advanced practice providers' performance based on facets of professional performance. The overall categories of practitioner, consultant, educator, researcher, and professional accountability from the advanced practice nurse (APN) position description were used for the evaluation. They initiated a workgroup of APNs and modified their standard categories to align with Benner's continuum from novice to expert and provided specific skills for each level to assist with the evaluation process. Feedback on using the tool was positive.

Managers often struggle with evaluating their direct care staff's practice, so Longo, Roussel, Pennington, and Hoying (2013) conducted a research study comparing the self-reported levels of expertise of staff nurses with the level of expertise identified by their managers. Data revealed that frontline clinical managers marked 73% of their direct reports at the same level of practicing RN as the individual's self identification. The same tool was used by both groups and included descriptions of the various levels of expertise.

The study by Specht (2013) used Benner's framework to identify successful role transition with novice faculty members. It explored the effects of mentoring on the levels of role conflict and role ambiguity experiences by novice nurse faculty related to their transitions into academe using a descriptive, comparative design. Results indicated that those who were mentored had lower levels of role conflict and role ambiguity than those who were not mentored.

Smith (2013) outlined implications for teaching strategies based on the five stages of skill acquisition. Benner's model of practice levels is significant because the degree of learning, based on knowledge and experience, has implications in structuring learning activities. The implications for teaching strategies based on the five stages of skill acquisition are included in Figure 4.2.

Figure 4.2 | Implications for Teaching Strategies Based on the Five Stages of Skill Acquisition

| Benner's skill level | Mode of inquiry | Type of learning (examples) | Learning experience/ methods (examples) |
|---|---|---|---|
| Novice | Basic instruction<br><br>Repeated guided practice | School of nursing basic prelicensure preparation<br><br>Teach rules, principles, concepts | Clinical component<br><br>Lab (skills and/or simulation)<br><br>Classroom<br><br>Precepted residency programs |

Figure 4.2 | Implications for Teaching Strategies Based on the Five Stages of Skill Acquisition (cont.)

| Benner's skill level | Mode of inquiry | Type of learning (examples) | Learning experience/ methods (examples) |
|---|---|---|---|
| Advanced beginner | Decrease instruction<br><br>Increase practice | Orientation to specific clinical specialty, including practice guidelines, policies, and professional standards<br><br>Socialization to work settings<br><br>Continuing education for information transmission<br><br>Core clinical programs | Unit orientation with preceptor to focus on aspect recognition in clinical practice and priority setting<br><br>Labs (skills and/or simulation)<br><br>Minimal formal classroom exposure<br><br>Networking: Who to go to for help |
| Competent | Primarily practice<br><br>Continuing education<br><br>Some inquiry | Continuing education for information transmission with application experiences and/ or problem solving<br><br>Update inservice programs<br><br>Decision-making games and situations that provide practice in planning and coordinating multiple complex assignments | Application component with more complexity<br><br>Simulations<br><br>Web-based courses<br><br>Networking |

Figure 4.2 | Implications for Teaching Strategies Based on the Five Stages of Skill Acquisition (cont.)

| Benner's skill level | Mode of inquiry | Type of learning (examples) | Learning experience/ methods (examples) |
|---|---|---|---|
| Proficient | Mainly practice<br><br>Self-directed learning<br><br>Increasing inquiry | Continuing education activities<br><br>Interdisciplinary conferences<br><br>Simulations<br><br>Case studies: Nurses identify interventions that made a positive difference and lessons learned<br><br>Learning: Cite examples and experiences<br><br>Inductive learning with nurse verbalizing his or her understanding of the situation | Application component with critical thinking<br><br>Networking to give help to others<br><br>Mentoring<br><br>Nursing rounds<br><br>Run simulations<br><br>Web-based courses |
| Expert | Practice inquiry<br><br>(Research) | Continuing education with a focus beyond institution<br><br>Research conferences<br><br>Peer review<br><br>Case presentations<br><br>Discussion and evaluation of observations with others<br><br>Clinical conferences that illustrate expertise | Serve as mentor<br><br>Clinical research<br><br>Application of research findings<br><br>Serve as model for competent and proficient nurses |

*Table developed by Kathleen J. Fischer (2009, p. 226); adapted by Charlene M. Smith, 2012. From Smith, C.M. (2013). Teaching learning methodologies. In S.L. Bruce (ed.), Core curriculum for nursing professional development. (4th ed., pp. 233–236). Chicago, IL: Association for Nursing Professional Development. Reprinted with permission.*

This chapter outlined the components of Benner's novice-to-expert theory, addressed strategies to transform nursing education, and included several examples of how Benner's model can be applied to practice.

# References

Benner, P. (1984). *From novice to expert: Excellence and power in clinical nursing practice.* Menlo Park, CA: Addison-Wesley.

Benner, P., Sutphen, M., Leonard, V., & Day, L. (2010). *Educating nurses: A call for radical transformation.* San Francisco, CA: Jossey-Bass.

Dole, J., Drews, B., Dimitt, P., Hildebrandt, E., Hittle, K., & Tielsch-Goddard, A. (2013). Novice to expert: The evolution of an advanced practice evaluation tool. *Journal of Pediatric Healthcare, 27*, 195–201.

George, J.B. (2011). *Nursing theories: The base for professional nursing practice.* 6th ed. Upper Saddle River, NJ: Pearson Education.

Gobet, F., & Chassy, P. (2008). Towards an alternative to Benner's theory of expert intuition in nursing: A discussion paper. *International Journal of Nursing Studies, 45*, 129–139. doi:10.1016/j.ijnurstu.2007.01.005.

Longo, M.A., Roussel, L., Pennington, S.L., & Hoying, C. (2013). The frontline clinical manager identifying direct reports' level of practice. *Journal of Pediatric Oncology Nursing, 30*, 260–268. doi:10.1177/1043454213493506.

Masters, K. (2012). *Nursing theories: A framework for professional practice.* Sudbury, MA: Jones and Bartlett Learning.

Smith, C.M. (2013). Teaching learning methodologies. In S.L. Bruce (ed.), *Core curriculum for nursing professional development* (4th ed., pp. 231–288). Chicago, IL: Association for Nursing Professional Development.

Specht, J.A. (2013). Mentoring relationships and the levels of role conflict and role ambiguity experienced by novice nursing faculty. *Journal of Professional Nursing, 29*, e25–e31. *http://dx.doi.org/10.1016/jprofnurs.2013.06.006.*

# Chapter 5

# Creating a Framework for Educator Competencies

| Learning Objective |
| --- |
| **After reading this chapter, the participant should be able to:** |
| ☑ Identify how the educational competencies fit with the nursing professional development (NPD) standards and Benner's novice-to-expert continuum |

The following definitions of key concepts from *Nursing Professional Development: Scope and Standards of Practice* (American Nurses Association [ANA] & National Nursing Staff Development Organization [NNSDO], 2010) are presented to guide the discussion in this chapter:

**Professional role competence:** Performance that meets defined criteria based on the specialty area, context, and model of practice in which an individual nurse is engaged.

**NPD specialist:** A registered nurse with expertise in nursing education who influences professional role competence and professional growth of nurses in a variety of settings, supports lifelong learning of nurses and other healthcare personnel in an environment that facilitates continuous learning, and fosters an appropriate climate for learning and facilitates the adult learning process.

**Standards of nursing practice:** Authoritative statements that describe a level of care or performance common to the profession of nursing by which the quality of nursing practice can be judged and reassured.

**Standards of professional performance:** Authoritative statements that describe a competent level of behavior in the professional role, including activities related to quality of NPD practice, education, professional practice evaluation, collegiality, collaboration, ethics, advocacy, research, resource utilization, and leadership.

# Framework

The NPD scope and standards of practice (ANA & NNSDO, 2010) can be used to provide a framework for the NPD competencies and performance criteria that were identified in the research studies. These standards are divided into nine standards of practice and 10 standards of professional performance.

Standards of practice:

1. Assessment

2. Identification of issues and trends

3. Outcomes identification

4. Planning

5. Implementation

    5a. Coordination

    5b. Learning and practice environment

    5c. Consultation

6. Evaluation

Standards of professional performance:

1. Quality of NPD practice

2. Education

3. Practice evaluation

4. Collegiality

5. Collaboration

6. Ethics

7. Advocacy

8. Research

9. Resource utilization

10. Leadership

The standards and corresponding outcome criteria focus on competencies appropriate for NPD specialists practicing in all settings.

# NPD Specialist Practice Model

The NPD standards are built upon a systems model that facilitates the professional development of nurses in their participation in lifelong learning activities to enhance their professional competence and role performance, the ultimate outcomes of which are protection of the public and the provision of safe, quality care (ANA & NNSDO, 2010). This process is illustrated with a systems model consisting of interrelated inputs, throughput, outputs, and feedback, as shown in Figure 5.1.

Figure 5.1 | Nursing Professional Development Specialist Practice Model

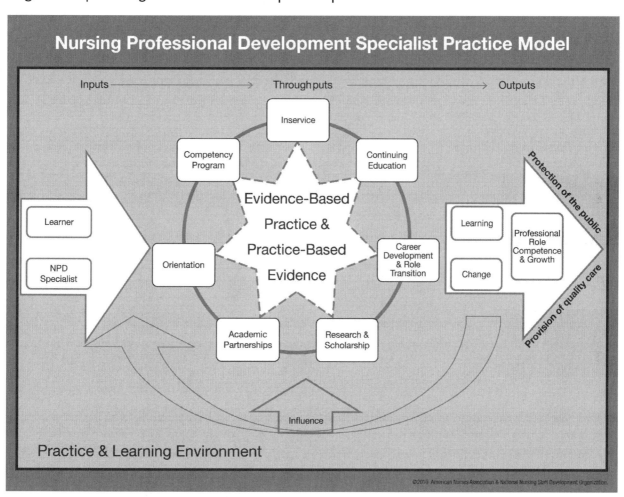

Source: Table from the American Nurses Association and National Nursing Staff Development Organization (2010) Scope and Standards of Practice for Nursing Professional Development. Washington, DC: American Nurses Publishing.

The model indicates that the provision of quality care and protection of the public are the ultimate outcomes of NPD practice, in addition to learning, change, and professional role competence and growth. The NPD specialist functions concurrently in both the practice environment and the learning environment. The practice environment supplies resources and creates the context that influences practice behaviors and outcomes, and the learning environment is any context in which learning occurs. These two environments have fluid boundaries and may intertwine at times.

The scope of responsibility and accountability for the NPD specialist evolves to meet the demands of the practice setting. Responsibilities for the functions listed below may vary based on the environment and type of NPD specialist position description:

- Career development responsibilities
- Education responsibilities
- Leadership responsibilities
- Program management responsibilities
- Compliance initiative responsibilities (ANA & NNSDO, 2010)

In the original *Scope and Standards for Nursing Professional Development* (ANA, 2000), six distinct roles were identified: educator, facilitator, change agent, consultant, leader, and researcher. These were the roles into which the competencies in the first edition of this book were put. However, the latest edition of the standards (ANA & NNSDO, 2010) recognized the complex nature of NPD practice and identified intertwined roles, which are:

- Educator/facilitator
- Educator/academic liaison
- Change agent/team member
- Researcher/consultant
- Leaders/communicator
- Collaborator/advisor/mentor

## What Was Done

The updated version of the competency assessment tool builds on the research study classifying the competencies into Benner's levels of expertise (Brunt, 2013). Initially, the author was going to place each of the competencies into the intertwined roles outlined in the latest edition of the standards. However, after asking a small group of six NPD experts to classify them into the intertwined elements, it became apparent that there was overlap, so the decision was made to keep them in Benner's level of expertise based on the feedback from participants in the research study. That feedback actually supported the concept that indeed the elements are intertwined. When the current NPD standards are revised, the format suggested by ANA is to use competency statements for each of the standards rather than the measurement criteria, as in the current standards. The workgroup that revises the standards can identify competencies for each of the standards.

For specific performance criteria for each of the statements, refer to the **Nursing Professional Development Specialist Competency Assessment Tool,** included in the appendix (you can download this tool, along with the rest of the resources, at *www.hcpro.com/downloads/12244)*. This tool has dark lines to differentiate the various levels of expertise but does not identify Benner's levels on the tool. Benner's model is situational, and it is recognized that the levels of expertise may vary based on one's individual role.

# Final List of Competencies by Category

The competencies listed are rank-ordered by level of expertise, with novice competencies listed first and progressing through the various stages to expert, based on the results from the research study. There were some competencies that did not seem to be classified in the appropriate level of expertise, but the results are presented based on the consensus of the 600-plus study participants. For instance, the competency "writes grant proposals or participates in the grant writing process" fell into the novice category, although that is not usually an expectation of a novice NPD educator. It could be the fact that since it had two verbs (both writing and participating) it was difficult to classify. The competency "facilitates change" was classified in the competent category, and in today's environment, this may be an expectation of a novice or advanced beginner educator.

**Novice** (mean 2.26–3.39)

1. Uses a variety of teaching strategies and audiovisuals
2. Promotes a safe and healthy work environment
3. Maintains confidentiality
4. Demonstrates expertise in use of computers
5. Maintains required documentation and record-keeping system
6. Provides technical assistance to clients
7. Maintains educational standards
8. Demonstrates proficiency in the use of technology
9. Writes grant proposals or participates in grant writing process
10. Integrates ethical principles in all aspects of practice
11. Maintains educational or clinical competencies appropriate for role
12. Promotes concept of lifelong learning

**Advanced beginner** (mean 3.4–3.59)

13. Participates in committees, task forces, projects, etc.
14. Develops or provides input into annual budget
15. Assists with excellence initiatives, such as Magnet® Recognition and Malcolm Baldrige National Quality Award
16. Involves the client in defining problems and selecting solutions
17. Establishes credibility with other professionals
18. Demonstrates emotional intelligence
19. Participates in activities external to practice setting

20. Networks within and outside nursing

21. Conducts focus groups

22. Accesses information external to organization

23. Assesses resources needed to facilitate research

24. Develops and conducts research

25. Facilitates the adult learning process, creating a climate conducive to learning and fostering a good relationship with learners

26. Identifies internal and external resources available for staff

27. Uses appropriate measurement tools and methods in quality improvement (QI) activities

28. Markets NPD and continuing education programs

29. Publishes information that can be used by other educators

**Competent** (mean 3.6-3.79)

30. Develops sponsor relationships with business and industry

31. Uses principles from theories of adult learning and organizational development, system change, and QI

32. Serves as a change agent

33. Uses appropriate measurement methods to assess and document competence of personnel

34. Communicates effectively with all levels of organization

35. Facilitates peer review

36. Facilitates change

37. Facilitates team-building

38. Functions within the political climate of the organization

39. Coaches and provides feedback to improve performance

40. Uses and evaluates materials resources and facilities

41. Conducts needs assessments using a variety of strategies

42. Critically processes information and problem-solves

43. Seeks opportunities to develop the various NPD intertwined elements of practice

44. Involves learners in assessment of needs and identification of outcomes

45. Demonstrates awareness of historical and emerging trends

46. Designs and revises educational activities

47. Serves as a role model for education

48. Supports integration of research into practice

49. Collaborates within and across organization

50. Develops links with academia and service

51. Ensures educational programs are congruent with organizational mission and goals

52. Communicates impact of new educational strategies to others

53. Produces desired outcomes relevant to organization

54. Interprets and communicates across boundaries

**Proficient** (mean 3.8–3.99)

55. Selects appropriate teaching strategies to facilitate behavioral change

56. Evaluates effectiveness and outcomes of educational endeavors

57. Incorporates research findings from a variety of disciplines into programs

58. Calculates risks and benefits of educational innovations

59. Creates and applies newer educational methodologies

60. Oversees evidence-based practice and practice-based evidence initiatives

61. Develops curricula (classes and courses around a common theme)

62. Evaluates overall program effectiveness

63. Consults on performance problems

64. Applies skill in strategic planning

65. Promotes career development and role transition

66. Maintains flexibility when managing multiple roles and responsibilities

67. Measures and communicates return on investment

68. Develops proactive educational policies and procedures for organization

69. Fosters systematic analysis of issues

70. Differentiates educational problems from system problems

71. Develops standards for educational practice in own setting

72. Sees beyond role-established boundaries

73. Determines and revises priorities for scheduled and unscheduled educational activities

**Expert** (mean 4.0–4.25)

74. Uses consultation skills internally and externally

75. Mentors other professionals

76. Incorporates transformational leadership principles into practice

77. Adjusts content and teaching strategies during presentation based on learners' reaction

78. Coordinates complex educational offerings

79. Possesses expert knowledge of how to teach within organizational culture.

*Source: ©2014 Barbara Brunt.*

To evaluate whether NPD educators are meeting the standards, outcome assessments can be used to identify, define, and communicate the skills and qualities that NPD educators should possess. Outcomes should be expressed in such a way that they:

- Reflect the vision of mission of the institution
- Are clear and unambiguous
- Are specific and address defined area of competence
- Are manageable in terms of the number of outcomes
- Are defined at an appropriate level of generality, assisting with the development of "enabling" outcomes
- Indicate the relationship between different outcomes

With the list of competencies provided, there are criteria for NPD specialists at any point on the continuum from novice-to-expert practitioner. Implementation of the competencies and corresponding performance criteria can be tailored to the individual's practice. This chapter described the framework for the competencies and the rationale for the ordering of competencies in each section. Practical application can be found in later chapters.

# References

American Nurses Association. (2000). *Scope and standards of practice for nursing professional development.* Washington, DC: American Nurses Publishing.

American Nurses Association and National Nursing Staff Development Organization. (2010). *Nursing professional development: Scope and standards of practice.* Silver Spring, MD: Nursesbooks.org.

Brunt, B.A. (2013). *Classifying nursing professional development competencies by level of expertise.* Unpublished research study.

# Chapter 6

# Methods to Validate Competencies

## How Do You Measure Competence?

There are numerous issues related to assessing and validating competence. Educators struggle with the following questions:

1. Who is responsible for assessing and documenting competence?

2. What tools can be used to validate competence?

3. How do you use competencies to evaluate performance?

4. How do you differentiate levels of competence?

Much of the discussion related to continued competence is focused on whose responsibility it is to assess and document competence. Most authors acknowledge individual responsibility and accountability. The American Nurses Association (ANA) Code of Ethics discusses the individual nurse's personal responsibility to maintain competence in practice (Fowler, 2008), and the ANA nursing scope and standards document reiterates the need for nurses to provide competent care and attain knowledge and competency that reflects current nursing practice. The scope and standards document for nursing professional development (NPD) is based on the concept of continuing competence (ANA and NNSDO, 2010).

The organization has a responsibility to ensure that all staff members providing patient care are appropriately educated and competent to fulfill their job responsibilities. Hospitals have an ethical and legal responsibility to make certain that the healthcare provided by its personnel meets acceptable standards. Employers carry out the requirements of The Joint Commission (TJC) and other accrediting bodies to ensure the ongoing competence of employees. Educators assist with this responsibility by developing competency assessment and/or development programs. NPD specialists often write competencies and validate both initial and continued competence.

Professional associations have a responsibility to set standards of performance and guidelines for safe practice. Competency validation is a partnership with the individual, agency, and professional association, as shown in Figure 6.1.

Figure 6.1 | Competency Validation Partnership

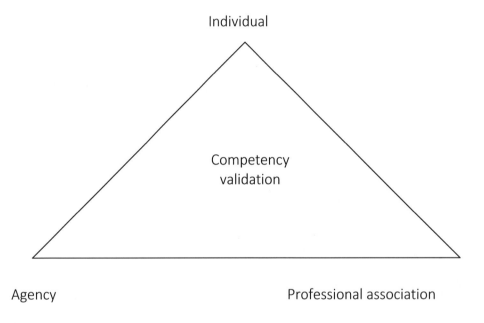

## Competency Checklists

Competency checklists are one way of validating competence. Checklists must clearly identify expectations and should be completed by staff members who know how to use them. Criteria for safe, effective performance must be clearly defined, and all participating in the evaluation process must have a common understanding of the criteria and the basis for assigning ratings. Research has shown that making direct observations using precise measurement criteria in checklists, with immediate feedback on performance, is more effective than the traditional evaluation of clinical skills using subjective rating forms. The format for skills checklists may vary, but most of them have similar information. Characteristics of competency checklists are identified in Figure 6.2.

Figure 6.2 | Characteristics of Competency Checklists

| |
|---|
| Learner oriented |
| Focus on behaviors |
| Measurable |
| Criteria validated by experts |
| Specific enough to avoid ambiguity |

Most checklists use a "met" and "not met" format, include an area for comments, and evaluate a single occurrence. One drawback with checklists is one does not know whether the observed behavior is a persistent one that is representative of the situation being observed, or whether it is a snapshot of performance at a particular point in time. It is also important to assess clinical competence in the context of the "real situation." Each institution determines how many and how often competency checklists should be used.

Some competency checklists have a self-assessment portion as part of the checklist. The self-assessment can give the evaluator an idea of the perceived skill level of the individual, although that can never take the place of validating the competency. Individuals may have different perceptions of their abilities, which may or may not be consistent with the evaluator's perceptions. For instance, some individuals could indicate they need practice, even though they are very familiar and competent with that skill, but they are not familiar with the institution's policy and procedure, while others could indicate they need practice because they have only done it once during their career. All required skills must be validated, regardless of the individual's assessment of his or her ability.

## Other Tools to Validate Competence

It is important to realize that there are numerous ways to validate competence. One of the most common ways is the competency checklist, but there are many other ways that competence can be validated (Wright, 2013, Brunt, 2008).

### Posttests

Posttests are one method to document cognitive knowledge and are sometimes used as a method to document competence. A posttest can be used to document basic knowledge so participants don't have to take a course or program when they can show they have the basic knowledge required in that course. For instance, some computer-based programs give participants the opportunity to complete the posttest first, and if they achieve a satisfactory score on the posttest, they don't have to complete the program. Tests can include a videotape or audiotape scenario, a live simulation, or printed or projected still pictures requiring a response from the individual. A crossword puzzle or word game can also serve as a posttest.

## Return demonstrations

Return demonstrations can either be done in artificial environments, such as in skills fairs or simulation labs, or in the real-world environment with one-on-one observations or bedside evaluation. The artificial environment provides an opportunity to practice the skill without creating any harm to patients.

## Case studies

Case studies can also be used to validate competence. Case studies are great for critical thinking and can reflect prioritization or problem solving. Most individuals are familiar with patient case studies, but these can be used for educational purposes also. Individuals could describe how they would provide education for a specific student or how they would deal with a particular scenario presented to them. See Figure 6.3 for an example of an educational case study.

Figure 6.3 | Sample Educational Case Study

**Situation:** You are teaching a mandatory session on a new model of care delivery to a large group of nurses at your institution. You have incorporated a variety of teaching strategies and an opening exercise to get everyone engaged in the topic. There is one learner who is being very vocal about not wanting to attend this session and questioning your ability to teach the content. The learner will not participate in the exercise and in front of the entire group loudly questions why this session is mandatory, as well as your authority to teach this.

1. What strategies can you use to deal with this difficult participant?
2. What adult learning strategies are appropriate for this situation?

## Simulations

Simulations, such as mock codes or demonstrating the skill on a simulation mannequin, can be used to validate competency. A room could be set up with a simulated patient who needed cardiopulmonary resuscitation or with numerous breaks in infection control techniques for participants to identify all the things that are not correct. Some schools use volunteers as simulated patients for staff to perform assessment or demonstrate various noninvasive clinical skills. Several companies have mannequins available that can simulate a variety of situations requiring interventions. There has been an increasing body of literature addressing various aspects of simulation from both the educational and practice perspectives. (Hagler & Wilson, 2013; Waterval, Stephen, Peczinka, & Shaw, 2012; McNeill, Parker, Nadeau, Pelaya, & Cook, 2012)

## Observations of daily work

Observations of daily work are another method of validating competence, often used in performance evaluations and with peer review or 360-degree evaluations. The 360-degree evaluation incorporates feedback from a variety of people who interact with an individual, including the manager, peers, individuals reporting to them, and so on. The use of different sources of information and different measures to evaluate competence increases validity.

# Competencies and Performance

Is there a difference between competence and performance? These terms are often used interchangeably in the literature. One way of differentiating these two concepts is to define competence as what a person knows and can do under ideal circumstances, while performance focuses on actual situated behavior—that is, what is actually done in the real-life context. If competence is causally related to performance, then the development of a competency should lead to increased effectiveness. However, one often observes a skill that is correlated with effective performance but that does not cause that performance.

For example, participants who are good at memorizing and writing may do well on tests, but that does not necessarily mean they will function more effectively in the clinical area. In developing training programs, the educator should remember that the employer judges competence of participants based on their ability to perform.

The goal of nursing education is to facilitate the transition of knowledge from the classroom to a variety of clinical experiences in a complex society with continually changing demographics, increased technology, and diminished resources. NPD specialists are challenged to use educational strategies to enhance student learning while also promoting clinical competency.

Meretoja and Koponen (2012) developed a three-step model to compare nurses' optimal and actual competencies in the clinical setting. The first component was the optimal competence profile, which included individual expert ratings and a group consensus profile. The second component was the actual competence profile, including the nurse ratings and nurse manager assessments. The third component was the educational challenges with the difference between the optimal and actual competence profiles and the continual learning culture and interventions.

Wilkinson (2013) did an integrative review of competency assessment tools for registered nurses and found four multidimensional research tools were used with nurses in ongoing practice. The tools specified a unique aspect on continuing competency, such as clinical care, leadership, and interpersonal relationship. Recognizing gaps in knowledge and the need for further research will assist the NPD specialist to evaluate the tools critically and could lead to the development of a more comprehensive assessment instrument.

# Differentiating Levels of Competence

Benner's work on differentiating levels of competence was described in Chapter 4. Although many authors have attempted to reflect differences in the level of practice, few have developed tools with specific criteria for each level. Levels of performance are often differentiated by the ability to analyze and synthesize information.

Case studies can be used to evaluate critical thinking skills, as well as open-ended questions to get feedback on thought processes.

Mind mapping and concept mapping are other strategies that may be used to identify and correlate multiple aspects of a concept or problem. Both of these formats are nonlinear outlines or graphic representations of concepts or problems. Learners begin by creating a colored image that represents the topic in the center of the paper. The next step is a "mind dump" in which participants write down all ideas related to the topic on a large piece of paper. Self-sticking notes may be used to jot down ideas and affix them to the paper. Participants can rearrange and cluster ideas in various configurations before settling on the most useful arrangement.

This chapter outlined various methods of validating competence and included information on whose responsibility it is to develop competence. Descriptions of various tools to document competence and a discussion of the difference between competence and performance were provided, as well as suggestions for ways to differentiate levels of competence.

# References

American Nurses Association and National Nursing Staff Development Organization. (2010). *Nursing professional development: Scope and standards of practice.* Silver Spring MD: Nursesbook.org.

Brunt, B.A. (2008). "What is competency validation?" In *Evidence-Based Competency Management System: A Toolkit for Validation and Assessment.* 2nd ed., pp. 21–39. Marblehead, MA: HCPro.

Fowler, M.D.M. (2008). *Guide to the code of ethics for nurses: Interpretation and application.* Silver Spring, MD: Nursesbooks.org.

Hagler, D., & Wilson, R. (2013). Designing nursing staff competency assessment using simulation. *Journal of Radiology Nursing,* 32(4), 165–169.

McNeill, J., Parker, R.A., Nadeau, J., Pelaya, L.W., & Cook, J. (2012). Developing nurse educator competency in the pedagogy simulation. *Journal of Nursing Education,* 51(12), 685–691. doi:10.3928/01484834-20121030-01.

Meretoja, R., & Koponen, L. (2012). A systematic model to compare nurses' optimal and actual competencies in the clinical setting. *Journal of Advanced Nursing,* 68(2), 412–422. doi: 10.1111/j.1365-2648.2011.05754.x.

Waterval, E.M.E., Stephen, K., Peczinka, D., & Shaw, A. (2012). Designing a process for simulation-based annual nurse competency assessment. *Journal for Nurses in Staff Development,* 28(6), 274–278. doi: 10.1097/NND.0b013e31827258f8.

Wilkinson, C.A. (2013). Competency assessment tools for registered nurses: An integrated review. *Journal of Continuing Education in Nursing,* 44(1), 31–37.

Wright, D. (2013). Competency programs. In S. L. Bruce, (ed.), *Core curriculum for nursing professional development* (4th ed, pp. 499–513). Chicago, IL: Association for Nursing Professional Development.

# Section II

# Applications of the Competencies to Practice

This section provides concrete examples of how the competencies can be used and applied in the practice setting in a variety of roles. Chapters include using the checklist as a self-assessment tool, using it to develop criterion-based position descriptions, using it to create an orientation for a new education, using it for performance appraisals/professional development plans, using it for a professional portfolio, and suggestions for documenting cultural competence. A new chapter was added on understanding generational differences.

# Chapter 7

# Self-Assessment Tool

| Learning Objective |
| --- |
| **After reading this chapter, the participant should be able to:** |
| ☑ Complete a self-assessment using the checklist |

Since the roles of nursing professional development (NPD) specialists vary based on the size and type of organization, competencies can be selected to accurately reflect the NPD role in various settings. All the competencies and performance criteria included in this book will not be applicable to all NPD specialists. Individuals can select the competencies that are appropriate for their current role and responsibilities. With the current emphasis on professional accountability, it is critical that NPD specialists, regardless of their role, demonstrate their competence and have a method to do so.

## Use as a Self-Assessment Tool

Wilkinson (2013) did an integrative review of the literature on self-assessment of continuing competence and found four research reports with multidimensional self-reporting tools designed to use with nurses in ongoing practice. The continuing competency of RNs is essential to their professional growth and confidence in the workplace. Understanding the importance and requirements of the continuing competency of RNs is the first task in choosing a self-reporting tool.

Practicing educators or individuals new to an educational role can use the tool provided in the appendix as a self-assessment. The tool provides an overview of all aspects of the educational role and can be tailored to the individual. For example, if an educator is in a setting that does not require research as part of the educational role, that competency can be ignored. Having specific

performance criteria identified for each competency can assist NPD specialists to determine if they have achieved
that competency.

The tool may also assist educators in identifying where they are on the novice-to-expert continuum. Since the competencies in each subcategory are ranked in order from novice to expert, educators who meet the competencies at the end of each role or category may be practicing at a more advanced level.

## Suggestions for using the self-assessment tool

**Questions to ask when completing a self-assessment:**

☑ Which of the skills are required in my current role or will be required in my new role?

☑ For each of those skills, can I provide examples of how I met the individual performance criteria?

☑ Are there some competencies where I met some but not all of the performance criteria listed?

☑ What experiences do I need to seek out to develop additional skills for a particular competency?

Information derived from the self-assessment can be private and does not need to be shared with others. The NPD specialist completing the self-assessment should answer the questions honestly and use the information obtained as a guide in seeking additional experiences to meet identified needs. Please note that even the most experienced educators will not be proficient in all the competencies listed. The number of competencies listed on the tool should not overwhelm new educators. This is designed as a tool to provide information for future learning opportunities.

# Reference

Wilkinson, C.A. (2013). Competency assessment tools for registered nurses: An integrative review. *The Journal of Continuing Education in Nursing,* 44(1), 31–3. *http://dx.doi.org/10.3928/00220124-20121101-53.*

# Chapter 8

# Developing Criterion-Based Position Descriptions

## Learning Objective

### After reading this chapter, the participant should be able to:

☑ Develop a nursing professional development (NPD) specialist position description specific to the setting

## Criterion-Based Position Descriptions

Many regulatory agencies, such as The Joint Commission, require organizations to have criterion-based position descriptions for staff, and the NPD competencies tool can be used to outline basic competencies and criteria included in a particular role.

Facilities can use the evidence-based data in the tool to write position descriptions. Since it provides a comprehensive classification of NPD competencies, it can be used for a variety of positions or in various settings. The roles and responsibilities of a one-person NPD department in a small hospital would be different than those of a 10-person NPD department in a large teaching hospital in a healthcare system. The competencies and criteria can be selected to fit multiples roles.

The qualifications for being an NPD specialist vary from setting to setting and are contingent on the roles and responsibilities of the department. There are various questions to consider before writing a position description, such as:

- What are the organization's philosophy, mission, vision, and values?
- Where does education fit within the organization?
- What are the goals and objectives of the education department?

- Is the organization a single entity or part of a larger healthcare system?

- What services does the education department provide (e.g., orientation, inservices, continuing education)?

- What are the reporting relationships?

- What educational qualifications are required for the position?

- What skills are required for the position?

- What is the organizational structure (e.g., centralized, decentralized, or a combination)?

According to Partington (2013), there are many practice settings for the NPD specialist outside of the acute care setting. These include ambulatory outpatient, community/public health, home health, and long-term care. Factors that impact the role of the NPD specialist in various settings include:

- Industry and professional standards

- Healthcare initiatives such as accountable care organizations, medical homes, and nurse-managed health centers

- Patient populations

- Resource management

- Workforce compensation

The structure of an education department will guide the development of position descriptions, since educators may function differently in centralized versus decentralized versus combination structures. In centralized models, NPD activities are performed by a core team of educators reporting to a single director. Decentralized models locate the responsibility for NPD at the level of the nursing department, a subdivision of that department, or at the unit level.

One form of a decentralized structure involves placing the responsibility for NPD within a central nursing administration, with educators assigned to specific roles. A second form may have some nurse educators assigned to a centralized NPD program and others attached to various clinical divisions with the nursing services department. The most extreme form of decentralization places all responsibilities for NPD on individual units.

Advantages and disadvantages of staff development structures are listed in Figure 8.1.

Figure 8.1 | Advantages and Disadvantages of Nursing Professional Development Structures

| | Advantages | Disadvantages |
|---|---|---|
| **Centralized** | Coordination of resources | Centralized decision-making |
| | Uniformity in implementing standards | Unresponsive to unit needs |
| | Coordination of regulatory and agency-required programming | Lack of coordination between general and unit programs |
| | Comprehensive and collaborative orientation activities | Lack of identity with specific areas |
| | Consistent education content and teaching methods | Dissatisfaction of educators with role |
| | More efficient use of educators | Possible reduced autonomy |
| | Support services readily available | Potential loss of clinical skills of educators |
| **Decentralized** | Educational needs more easily identified | Coordination may be ineffective or inefficient |
| | Increased opportunity for feedback and application | Duplication of education and efforts of personnel |
| | Increased educational leadership and involvement in departments | Inconsistent education and teaching methods |
| | Programming implemented in a timely manner | Lack of support services |
| | More flexibility in educational programming | Inadequate or inconsistent record keeping |
| | Educators seen as clinical experts | Educators may be used for service |
| **Combination** | Identification of individual unit needs | Cost of managing both designs may increase staffing |
| | Timely response to both centralized and decentralized education | Educators may lose sight of overall staff development goals |
| | Use of clinical experts for unit-based programming | |
| | Increased flexibility | |
| | Availability of support services | |
| | Coordination to reduce duplication and inappropriate use of resources | |
| | Collegial support for all educators | |

*Source: ©1998 Lippincott, Williams & Wilkins. Brunt, B. "Structure and process: New models of nursing and clinical staff development." In K. J. Kelly-Thomas. Clinical and Nursing Staff Development: Current Competence, Future Focus. 2nd ed. Philadelphia: Lippincott Williams & Wilkins. Reproduced with permission.*

Once the questions are answered, then the competencies can be used as a framework to either develop the position descriptions or ensure that the essential competencies are identified in the position descriptions. Sample position descriptions for a nursing professional development educator, director of nursing research and professional development, and system director for employee development are included as Exhibits 8.1, 8.2, and 8.3.

> TIP: Develop position descriptions to include specific competencies/expectations in the educator/administrator role in your setting.

# References

Brunt, B. (1998). Structure and process: New models of nursing and clinical staff development. In K.J. Kelly-Thomas, *Clinical and nursing staff development Current competence, future focus* (2nd ed. pp. 25–53). Philadelphia: Lippincott Williams & Wilkins.

Partington, B. (2013). Role of the nursing professional development specialist in various health care settings. In S.L. Bruce (ed.), *Core curriculum for nursing professional development*. (4th ed., pp. 319–335). Chicago, IL: Association for Nursing Professional Development.

Summa Health System. (2013). Position Description for Nursing Professional Development Educator. Akron, OH: Author.

Summa Health System. (2012). Position Description for Director of Nursing Research and Professional Development. Akron, OH: Author.

Summa Health System. (2014). Position Description for System Director of Employee Development. Akron, OH: Author.

Exhibit 8.1 | Nursing Professional Development Job Description

# Anytown Health System

# Nursing Professional Development Job Description

**Job Title:** Nursing Professional Development Educator

**Reports to:** Director, Nursing Research and Professional Development

**Indirectly Reports to:** Unit Director, other VP's of Patient Care and Clinical Services

**Department:** Nursing Professional Development

**Date:** _____

**Written by:** _____

FLSA Status: Exempt

## Summary of Position

Designs, organizes, implements, and evaluates educational programs (orientations, continuing education, and inservices) that facilitate the professional growth, skill development, competency, and attainment of standards of care for direct care providers within the following departments: Department of Patient Care Services and Ambulatory Care Services.

## Minimum Qualifications

- Formal education required:
  - Current license to practice nursing
  - Master's degree in nursing or education OR
  - Baccalaureate degree in nursing and currently enrolled in master's degree program

- Experience and training required:
  - Three (3) years professional RN experience
  - One (1) year formal teaching experience

- Other skills, competencies, and qualifications:
  - Excellent verbal and written communication skills

### Exhibit 8.1 | Nursing Professional Development Job Description (cont.)

- Ability to work collaboratively with various levels of nursing personnel, medical staff, community representatives
- Ability to use computer and audiovisual equipment

- **Population-specific competency:**
  - Ability to effectively interact with populations of patients/customers with an understanding of their needs for self-respect and dignity

- **Level of physical demands:**
  - Medium: Exerts 20–50 pounds of force occasionally and/or 10–25 pounds of force frequently, and/or a negligible amount of force continuously to move objects

## Essential Functions

The following job-specific requirements should discuss the <u>essential</u> duties and responsibilities required of the position. They should not replicate those duties and responsibilities discussed above.

1. **Orientation**
   - Plans, organizes, implements, and evaluates clinical orientation for all levels of nursing personnel both at the individual and departmental levels.

2. **Policy and Procedure Writing**
   - Writes and revises the Department of Patient Care Services policies and procedures utilizing nursing theory. Assists nursing units to write and revise their department/unit policies and procedures.

3. **Continuing Education**
   - Writes continuing nursing education (CE) applications for selected educational programs following the Ohio Nurses Association CE Providership Guidelines and by the knowledge of basic nursing principles based on the biological, physical, and psycho-social sciences.

4. **BLS/ACLS/Crisis Intervention, Neonatal Resuscitation, and Fetal Monitoring**
   - Prepares and teaches in the mandatory BLS/ACLS/Crisis Intervention, Neonatal Resuscitation, and Fetal Monitoring courses.

5. **Consultation**
   - Prepares and/or assists clinical nursing personnel to work with other members of the healthcare team to care for/teach patients/populations of patients focusing on clear communication and constructive feedback to achieve healthcare goals.

## Exhibit 8.1 | Nursing Professional Development Job Description (cont.)

### 6. Curriculum/Inservices

- Collaborates with nursing managers, nursing staff peers, and other hospital departments; designs, organizes, implements and evaluates curriculums and in-services that assist nursing personnel to care for various populations of patients with the goal of attaining, maintaining, and restoring optimum health.

Note: The above-stated duties are intended to outline those functions typically performed by the incumbent in this position. This description of duties is not intended to be all-inclusive or to limit the discretionary authority of supervisors to assign additional tasks of a similar nature or level of responsibility.

*Source: Summa Health System. (2013). Position Description for Nursing Professional Development Educator. Akron, OH: Author. Reprinted with permission.*

## Exhibit 8.2 | Director, Nursing Research and Professional Development

# Anytown Health System
# Management job description

**Job Title:** Director, Nursing Research and Professional Development
**Department:** Nursing Professional Development
**Date:** _____
**Written by:** _____

## Summary of Position

Facilitates, directs, and coordinates the designing, planning, implementing, and evaluating of educational programs, activities, and services for the Department of Patient Care Services and Ambulatory Care Services. Ensures that such programs/services promote professional growth of personnel, competency of personnel, learning needs of patients and families, and attainment of hospital's strategic goals. Ensures that educational programs/services are consistent with criteria and standards of care established by licensing and accrediting bodies and professional organizations with the goal of attaining, maintaining, and restoring optimum health. Coordinates orientations/clinical experiences for all graduate nursing students coming to Anytown Health System. Coordinates tracking of hospitalwide educational/safety programs. Oversees nursing research and clinical nurse specialists.

## Dimensions of Position

Operating budget:
    Revenue: $11,000
          Expenses: $1,281,704

## Minimum Qualifications

Formal education required:

- BSN with master's degree or MSN
- Certification preferred—or required to obtain within two (2) years

Experience and training required:

- Five (5) years related professional experience
- Two (2) years in a supervisory or management position

## Exhibit 8.2 | Director, Nursing Research and Professional Development (cont.)

Other skills, competencies, and qualifications:

- Ability to direct the work effort of others through teamwork and building
- Ability to communicate verbally and in writing with physicians, hospital staff, educational institution representatives and professional group representatives
- Ability to assess, implement, and evaluate educational needs and programs designed to meet needs of staff, patients, families, physicians, and nursing and allied health students
- Ability to work collaboratively with nursing personnel, physicians, hospital departments, and community institutions' representatives
- Ability to use computer and audiovisual equipment
- Ability to manage multiple projects at one time
- Population-specific competency: Ability to effectively interact with patients/customers with the understanding of their needs for self-respect and dignity

Level of physical demands:

- **Medium:** Exerts 20–50 pounds of force occasionally and/or 10–25 pounds of force frequently, and/or a negligible amount of force continuously to move objects

# Direct Management Reporting Relationships

Indicate the title that this position reports to, as well as the various titles reporting directly to this position. *Include FTE counts.*

**Position reports to**: CNO/VP Patient Care Services

**Positions reporting to this position**:
*Note: This includes FTEs over which this position has hire, fire, and performance review responsibilities.*

Total FTEs: 17.3

- 79151 Staff Development Instructors
- 79181 Support Specialists and Senior Administrative Secretaries
- 75611 Coordinator of Educational Facilities
- 69051 Virtual Care Stimulation Lab Coordinator and Secretary
- 52240 Nursing Research Coordinator
- 69011 Advanced Practice Nurses

---

### Exhibit 8.2 | Director, Nursing Research and Professional Development (cont.)

# Key Results & Accountability Areas:

The following key results and accountability areas will be carried out in a manner fully consistent with the Anytown Health System mission, values, and philosophies.

1. **Financials**

   ■ Plans, prepares, implements, and monitors area's operational and capital budgets to ensure sound fiscal management consistent with the goals of Anytown Health System.

   ■ Manages productivity within department; minimum target is 100%; meets targets set in assigned area.

2. **Managing & Leading People**

   ■ Manages performance and ensures 100% of all required performance appraisals are completed.

   ■ Ensures all staff members complete Mandatory Organizational Education (MOE) training annually.

   ■ Ensures all staff members adhere to established Service Excellence Standards.

   ■ Monitors and manages staffing, turnover, and vacancy in assigned departments.

   ■ Ensures continued development and education of self and staff.

   ■ Ensures excellent open communications within the department through regular staff meetings, preparation and distribution of minutes, and other means to keep the department informed on a timely basis.

3. **Service Excellence**

   Identifies the direct and indirect groups served by assigned department, determining appropriate products and/or services based upon groups' served needs, measuring group's satisfaction and developing actions that continually improve services. Ensures staff and self work to achieve service excellence to the fullest extent possible. Groups served may include patients, visitors, employees, managers, vendors and/or physicians.

4. **Planning & Organizing**

   Plans and organizes all activities under his/her control in an effective manner. Prepares departmental tactical and strategic plans as well as designing appropriate organizational structures for areas of responsibility. Organizes and delegates work in an effective manner, establishes appropriate time frames for completion of work, and provides the necessary leadership to ensure effective work results.

---

## Exhibit 8.2 | Director, Nursing Research and Professional Development (cont.)

### 5. <u>Performance Improvement</u>

Ensures that his/her department adopts a Total Quality Improvement approach to its work that includes employee empowerment, managing with data, a philosophy of continual improvement, a customer-driven attitude, and a work methodology that maximizes error prevention. Develops and maintains a complete quality monitoring system throughout their department.

### 6. <u>Relationships with Managers, Peers, etc.</u>

Develops and maintains open, honest, and mutually beneficial relationships with their manager, fellow managers, staff and the departments to which he/she provides service. Relationships will be maintained in a manner consistent with Anytown Health System's mission, values, and philosophies.

### 7. <u>Support Diversity</u>

Ensures a work environment that promotes and embraces diversity. Works to support and strengthen Anytown Health System's service to the community.

### 8. <u>Regulatory Compliance</u>

- Complies with regulatory and accreditation requirements through completion of Anytown Health System's mandatory organizational education, TJC, Code of Conduct, and compliance training. Responsible for adherence to applicable regulations in daily activities and work processes.

- Supports strategic hospital goals by providing clerical support to all departments, by the running of compliance statistics for Mandatory Organizational Education and Code of Conduct, BLS/ACLS stats, employee educational records for performance appraisals, and providing student and guest housing facilities.

### 9. <u>Additional Job Specific Duties:</u>

The following key results and accountability areas should be specific to this position. There should be major categories of responsibility and measures of accountability and expectations included for each major category. Note these areas of responsibility should not duplicate those previously covered above.

### 1. **Education Programs/Services for Department of Patient Care Services**

- Facilitates orientations, curriculums, inservices, professional community workshops, mandatory BLS/ACLS/NPR/NVCI programs, and competency system for direct patient care providers. Teaches in selected programs.  Oversees nursing research and clinical nurse specialists.

## Exhibit 8.2 | Director, Nursing Research and Professional Development (cont.)

**2. Continuing Education**

- Oversees continuing nursing education (CE) application system for selected educational programs following the State Nurses Association's CE Providership Guidelines and by the knowledge of basic nursing principles based on the biological, physical and psycho-social sciences.

**3. Policy and Procedure Writing**

- Oversees the writing and revising of the Department of Patient Care Services policies and procedures

- BLS/ACLS/Crisis Intervention, Neonatal Resuscitation and Fetal Monitoring
  - Oversees mandatory BLS/ACLS/Crisis Intervention, Neonatal Resuscitation, and Fetal Monitoring courses. Teaches BLS.

- Patient Education
  - Ensures a system that assists clinical nursing personnel to develop/purchase materials to teach patients/populations of patients focusing on clear communication and constructive feedback to achieve healthcare goals.

- Affiliating Clinical Rotations
  - Collaborates with the colleges and universities of nursing to provide educational clinical experiences/activities of mutual concern/need.

Note: The above-stated duties are intended to outline those functions typically performed by the incumbent in this position. This description of duties is not intended to be all-inclusive or to limit the discretionary authority of supervisors to assign additional tasks of a similar nature or level of responsibility.

*Source: Summa Health System. (2012). Position Description for Director, Nursing Research and Professional Development. Akron, OH: Author. Reprinted with permission.*

---

Exhibit 8.3 | System Director of Employee Development

# Anytown Health System
# Management job description

Job Title: System Director of Employee Development

Department: Human Resources

Date: _____

Written by: _____

## Summary of Position

Provides overall leadership for clinical and nonclinical employee education and development including the designing, planning, implementing, and evaluation of employee educational programs, activities, and services for Summa Health System. Establishes and implements a strategic plan for employee development that fulfills the current and future workforce needs of the organizations. Ensures that programs/services promote professional growth of personnel, competency of staff, and learning needs that support Summa Health System's strategic goals. Ensures that educational programs/services are consistent with criteria and standards of care established by licensing and accrediting bodies and professional organizations with the goal of attaining, maintaining, and restoring optimum health. Directs tracking of hospitalwide educational/safety programs.

## Dimensions of Position

Operating Budget:

- Revenue:
- Expenses:

## Minimum Qualifications

Formal education required:

- BSN with master's degree in related field
- Ohio RN license

Experience and training required:

- Five (5) + years related professional experience in the field of employee development and learning

---

## Exhibit 8.3 | System Director of Employee Development (cont.)

- Five (5) + years in a leadership role

Other skills, competencies, and qualifications:

- Ability to direct the work effort of others through teamwork and consensus building
- Ability to communicate verbally and in writing with internal customers, educational institution representatives, and professional group representatives
- Ability to assess, implement, and evaluate educational needs and programs designed to meet needs of staff, patients, families, as well as nursing and allied health students
- Ability to work collaboratively with nursing personnel, physicians, hospital departments, and community institutions' representatives
- Ability to use computer and audiovisual equipment
- Ability to manage multiple projects at one time
- Population-specific competency: Ability to effectively interact with patients/customers with the understanding of their needs for self-respect and dignity

Level of physical demands:

- **Sedentary:** Exerts up to ten pounds of force occasionally and/or a negligible amount of force frequently.

# Direct Management Reporting Relationships

Indicate the title which this position reports to, as well as the various titles reporting directly to this position. *Include FTE counts.*

**Position reports to:** Senior VP, Human Resources

**Positions reporting to this position:**

- Administrative Secretary (1 FTE)
- Coord, Educational Facilities (1 FTE)
- Coord, Simulation Lab (1 FTE)
- Health Educator WRH (0.6 FTE)
- HRD Instructor (0.8 FTE)
- Instructional Developer (1 FTE)
- Leadership Development Coach (0.8 FTE)
- NPD Educator (6.1 FTE)
- Nursing Education Support Spec (1 FTE)

## Exhibit 8.3 | System Director of Employee Development (cont.)

- Secretary (0.5 FTE)
- Staff Development Instructor (2.8 FTE)

*Note: This includes FTEs over which this position has hire, fire, and performance review responsibilities.*

# Essential Functions

The following essential functions will be carried out in a manner fully consistent with the Anytown Health System mission, values, and philosophies.

1. **Financials**

   - Plans, prepares, implements, and monitors area's operational and capital budgets to ensure sound fiscal management consistent with the goals of Anytown Health System.
   - Manages productivity within the department; minimum target is 100%; meets targets set in assigned area.

2. **Managing & Leading People**

   - Manages performance and ensures 100% of all required performance appraisals are completed.
   - Ensures all staff members complete Mandatory Organizational Education (MOE) training annually.
   - Ensures all staff members adhere to established Service Excellence Standards.
   - Monitors and manages staffing, turnover and vacancy in assigned departments.
   - Ensures continued development and education of self and staff.
   - Ensures excellent open communications within the department through regular staff meetings, preparation, and distribution of minutes, and other means to keep the department informed on a timely basis.
   - Manages multiple cost centers, to include Nursing Professional Development Educational Facilities, Nursing Education, Virtual Care Simulation Lab, Education and Staff Development, HR Development, etc., and multiple foundation accounts.

3. **Service Excellence**

   Identifies the direct and indirect customers served by assigned department, determining appropriate products and/or services based upon customers' needs, measuring customers satisfaction, and developing actions that continually improve services.

## Exhibit 8.3 | System Director of Employee Development (cont.)

Ensures staff and self follow Service Excellence Standards of Behavior, including standards for Appearance and Environment, Attitude and Courtesy, Communication, Teamwork, Customer Service, Confidentiality, Safety, and Etiquette.

### 4. <u>Planning & Organizing</u>

Plans and organizes all activities under his/her control in an effective manner. Prepares departmental tactical and strategic plans as well as designing appropriate organizational structures for areas of responsibility. Organizes and delegates work in an effective manner, establishes appropriate time frames for completion of work, and provides the necessary leadership to ensure effective work results.

Facilitates, directs, and coordinates the designing, planning, implementing, and evaluation of educational programs, activities, and services for Anytown Health System personnel.

### 5. <u>Performance Improvement</u>

Ensures that his/her department adopts a Total Quality Improvement approach to its work that includes employee empowerment, managing with data, a philosophy of continual improvement, a customer-driven attitude, and a work methodology that maximizes error prevention. Develops and maintains a complete quality monitoring system throughout their department.

### 6. <u>Relationships with Managers, Peers, etc.</u>

Develops and maintains open, honest, and mutually beneficial relationships with their manager, fellow managers, staff, and the departments to which he/she provides service. Maintains relationships in a manner consistent with Anytown Health System's mission, values, and philosophies.

- Collaborates with other leaders for development and revision of appropriate policies and procedures
- Collaborates with clinical leaders to coordinate education and training provided through department-level educators/trainers to ensure efficient use of resources and quality of education and training provided throughout the system

### 7. <u>Supports Diversity and Community</u>

Ensures a work environment that promotes and embraces diversity. Works to support and strengthen Anytown Health System's service to the community.

### 8. <u>Regulatory Compliance</u>

Complies with regulatory and accreditation requirements through completion of Anytown Health System's mandatory organizational education, TJC, Code of Conduct, and compliance training. Responsible for adherence to applicable regulations in daily activities and work processes.

Exhibit 8.3 | System Director of Employee Development (cont.)

- Ensures adherence to State Board of Nursing and ANCC standards for continuing nursing education (CE) programs

## Additional Job Duties (note these areas of responsibility should not duplicate those previously covered above)

1. Assess educational needs of personnel in order to plan effective education and development. Ensures that educational programs/services promote professional growth and competency of personnel and attainment of Anytown Health System's strategic plan. Coordinates preceptor education. Teaches selected programs.

2. Ensures that educational programs/services are consistent with criteria and standards of care established by licensing and accrediting bodies and professional organizations with the goal of attaining, maintaining, and restoring optimum health and patient safety.

3. Collaborates with educational institutions to foster educational opportunities/experiences for students and others interested in healthcare. Oversees the coordination of student nurse clinical rotations in southwest region only along with systemwide clinical rotations for medical assistants, physician assistants, nurse practitioners, etc.

4. Collaborates with other leaders on the team in support of workforce development and planning by supporting or directing workforce readiness programs such as NEONI, HIP, Project Search, etc.

5. Manages online learning management system, including assignments, creation of groups, and tracking compliance with mandatory education.

6. Facilitates new employee orientation and clinical orientation curriculum, inservices, professional community workshops, mandatory BLS/ACLS/NRP/NVCI programs, and competency assessment system.

7. Ensures nonclinical education including tuition reimbursement, Anytown Health System's Learning Center, and other education offerings are in support of Anytown Health System's strategic plan.

8. Oversees selected patient/family education processes.

9. Oversees Anytown Health System scholarship programs.

10. Ensures educational representation on committees systemwide and/or personally attends meetings.

*Note: The above-stated duties are intended to outline those functions typically performed by the incumbent in this position. This description of duties is not intended to be all-inclusive or to limit the discretionary authority of supervisors to assign additional tasks of a similar nature or level of responsibility.*

*Source: Summa Health System. (2014). Position Description for System Director of Employee Development. Akron, OH: Author. Reprinted with permission.*

# Chapter 9

# Orientations for New Educators

## Orientation for New Educators

Administrators or institutions can use the tool to plan an orientation program for a new NPD specialist. Specific job expectations and competencies can be identified, and the performance criteria can be used to plan experiences to meet those expectations. Since the competencies are categorized by the roles identified in the American Nurses Association and National Nursing Staff Development Organization (2010) standards for NPD, experiences relating to various aspects of the educational role can be included.

Orientations should focus on evidence-based practice (EBP) in NPD. EBP involves an ongoing analysis of NPD practice for the purpose of identifying those NPD interventions that best facilitate learning and enhance job performance. Plan your orientation starting with a determination of the practitioner's level of expertise and the NPD competencies that must be achieved. Areas that should be addressed within the orientation include:

- Needs assessment
- Planning
- Implementation
- Program evaluation

- Resistant learners
- Inservice education
- Committee membership (Avillion & Buchwald, 2010)

With individuals new to an educational role, the emphasis should be on the educator competencies rather than some of the other roles, but the orientation can be tailored to meet the needs of the individual educator. If the individual educator completes the tool as a self-assessment prior to the orientation, the orientation can be planned to ensure that the educator gains experience in areas of identified needs.

Figure 9.1 shows how an orientation program could be established using these competencies.

### Figure 9.1 | Example of an Orientation Program Based on Selected Roles

| Category and competency | Resources/experiences to meet competency |
|---|---|
| Educator/Facilitator: Designs and revises education activities | - Review materials on adult learning principles<br>- Read Chapters 9 and 13 in *Core Curriculum*<br>- Observe planning and implementation of educational program<br>- View video on teaching adults |
| Educator/Facilitator: Uses a variety of teaching strategies and audiovisuals | - Spend time with media expert or experienced educator to learn about AV equipment/resources<br>- Read Chapters 10 and 23 in *Core Curriculum*<br>- Review AV design information |
| Educator/Facilitator: Conducts needs assessment using a variety of strategies | - Read Chapter 8 in *Core Curriculum*<br>- Review completed needs assessments, results, and communication strategies<br>- Complete needs assessment for one area of responsibility |
| Educator/Facilitator: Identifies internal and external resources available for staff | - Review chapter 13 in *Core Curriculum*<br>- Spend time with another educator to identify internal resources<br>- Identify resources on the Internet<br>- Gather information about professional organizations with an educational component or focus |

Figure 9.1 | Example of an Orientation Program Based on Selected Roles (cont.)

| Category and competency | Resources/experiences to meet competency |
|---|---|
| Educator/Academic Liaison: Develops links with academia and service | - Review Chapter 32 of *Core Curriculum*<br>- Discuss role of nurses in precepting nursing students with clinical faculty<br>- Work collaboratively with academia to further service priorities<br>- Serve as adjunct faculty at a local college or university, if appropriate |
| Change agent/team member: Serves as a change agent | - Review Chapter 31 in *Core Curriculum*<br>- Work with colleague on a change project<br>- Assist with evaluation of the impact of change<br>- Promote problem solving by clarifying issues related to change project |
| Researcher/Consultant: Participates in committees, task forces, projects, etc. | - Observe various committee meetings<br>- Work with colleagues on a group project<br>- Watch video on conducting effective meetings<br>- Develop agenda for a meeting |
| Researcher/Consultant: Supports integration of research into practice | - Review evidence-based practice and practice-based evidence information<br>- Review Chapter 30 in *Core Curriculum*<br>- Incorporate current research data into a presentation and own practice<br>- Encourage critical thinking<br>- Develop information to assist staff evaluate research articles |
| Leader/Communicator: Maintains required documentation and record-keeping system | - Review Chapter 19 in *Core Curriculum*<br>- Read record-keeping policies and procedures for department<br>- Review continuing education files/reports<br>- Complete file for program taught |

Figure 9.1 | Example of an Orientation Program Based on Selected Roles (cont.)

| Category and competency | Resources/experiences to meet competency |
|---|---|
| Leader/Communicator: Maintains confidentiality and integrates ethical principles in all aspects of practice | - Review organizational policies and procedures on confidential information<br>- Review Chapter 27 in *Core Curriculum*<br>- Do not include identifying information on class materials or in presentation |
| Collaborator/Advisor/Mentor: | - Review Chapter 34 in *Core Curriculum*<br>- Meet with key stakeholders/individuals to better understand their role in the organization<br>- Identify opportunities for staff to increase skill and competence<br>- Seek out mentor for education |

Reference: Bruce, S.L. (ed.) (2013). *Core curriculum for nursing professional development.* (4th ed). Chicago, IL: Association for Nursing Professional Development.

Another format that could be used for an orientation program is provided in Exhibit 9.1.

Exhibit 9.1 | Sample Orientation Schedule for New Medical/Surgical Educator

# Anytown Health System Nursing Education and Staff Development

## Orientation for Medical-Surgical Educator

## Week 1

| | | |
|---|---|---|
| **Monday, July 4** | PTO | |
| Tuesday, July 5 | | |
| 8:00–8:30 A.M. | Welcome—get keys and settled into office | Room 233 |
| 8:30 –11:00 A.M. | Meet with Staff Development Director regarding: | Director's Office |

Mission, Philosophy, Objections of Department
Organization
Overview of Programs
Resources:     Phone list
                   Clinical descriptions
                   Monthly calendar
                   Staff development core curriculum

| | | |
|---|---|---|
| 11:00–12:00 P.M. | Lunch with all the staff development instructors | |
| 12:00–1:00 P.M. | Meet with critical care educator regarding: | Room 232 |

CCENC
____ Conference
PV Workshop

| | | |
|---|---|---|
| 1:00–2:00 P.M. | Meet with education facilities coordinator regarding: | Education coordinator's Office |

Room/AV Requests
Building Issues

## Exhibit 9.1 | Sample Orientation Schedule for New Medical/Surgical Educator (cont.)

| Time | Activity | Location |
|------|----------|----------|
| 2:00–3:00 P.M. | Meet with administrative secretary regarding:<br>Supplies<br>Typing requests<br>Time requests<br>Voice mail<br>Email<br>Registration process | SD Office |
| 3:00–4:00 P.M. | Meet with behavioral health educator regarding:<br>NA Orientation<br>US Orientation<br>Behavioral Health Workshop | Room 228 |
| 4:00–4:30 P.M. | Catch-up/review information for the day | |

**Wednesday, July 6**

| Time | Activity | Location |
|------|----------|----------|
| 8:00–9:00 A.M. | Catch-up: emails/voice mails | |
| 9:00–10:00 A.M. | Meet with patient education coordinator regarding:<br>Patient education<br>Ambulatory Workshop | Room 230 |
| 10:00–11:00 A.M. | Meet with medical librarian<br>Orientation to medical library | Medical Library |
| 11:00–12:00 P.M. | Lunch | |
| 12:00N–1:00 P.M. | Meet with OB educator regarding:<br>NRP, all OB Courses/Workshops | Room 227 |
| 1:00–2:00 P.M. | Meet with media services specialists<br>Media services, AV equipment, posters | Media–PCS Ground |
| 2:00–3:00 P.M. | Meet with nursing resources re: orientation<br>hiring process | Nsg Office Conf Rm |
| 3:00–4:00 P.M. | Meet with unit manager | 5 North Manager's Office |
| 4:00–4:30 P.M. | Catch-up | |

## Exhibit 9.1 | Sample Orientation Schedule for New Medical/Surgical Educator (cont.)

**Thursday, July 7**

| | | |
|---|---|---|
| 8:00–9:00 A.M. | Meet with simulation specialist re: simulations | VCSL (Sim Lab) |
| 9:00–10:00 A.M. | Meet with unit manager | 4 North Manager's Office |
| 10:00–11:30 A.M. | Meet with administrative director's M/S C/C leadership group | Dining Room A |
| 11:30–12:30 P.M. | Lunch | |
| 12:30–1:00 P.M. Room 233 | Emails/Voice mails, etc. | |
| 1:00–2:00 P.M. | Meet with surgical services educators Surgical services orientation/education | Office in OR area |
| 2:00–3:00 P.M. | Meet with Unit Manager | 6 East Manager's Office—6 East |
| 3:00–4:00 P.M. | Meet with Unit Manager | 6 West Manager's Office |
| 4:00 – 4:30 P.M. | Catch-up before leaving for PTO | |

| | |
|---|---|
| **Friday, July 8** | Preapproved PTO |

# Week 2

**Monday, July 11**

Attend Nursing Professional Development Leadership Council meeting in the morning (CR 2 8:00–11:00 A.M.) and meet with _____ about orientation in the afternoon

---

**Exhibit 9.1 | Sample Orientation Schedule for New Medical/Surgical Educator (cont.)**

**Tuesday, July 12**

| | | |
|---|---|---|
| 7:30 –4:00 P.M. | Sit through RN/LPN orientation | Classroom D |

**Wednesday, July 13**

| | | |
|---|---|---|
| 8:00–5:00 P.M. | Sit through RN/LPN orientation | Classroom D/Annex 4 Classroom |

**Thursday, July 14**

| | | |
|---|---|---|
| 8:00–5:00 P.M. | Sit through RN/LPN orientation | Classroom D/Annex 4 Classroom |

**Friday, July 15**

| | | |
|---|---|---|
| 8:00 - 4:00 P.M. | Sit through RN/LPN orientation | Classroom D |

## Week 3

**Monday, July 18**

| | | |
|---|---|---|
| 7:30–8:00 A.M. | Emails, voice mail | |
| 8:00 –4:00 P.M. | Sit through RN/LPN orientation | Classroom B |

**Tuesday, July 19**

| | | |
|---|---|---|
| 8:00–10:00 A.M. | Catch-up, organize information to date | |
| 10:00–11:00 A.M. | Meet with Director regarding:<br>CE system/forms<br>Policy/Procedure System<br>Clinical Rotation Schedule<br>Nursing Student Tech Orientation | Director's Office |
| 11:00–12:00 P.M. | Lunch | |
| 12:00 -4:00 P.M. | Med-surg curriculum—day 1 | Classroom D |

---

## Exhibit 9.1 | Sample Orientation Schedule for New Medical/Surgical Educator (cont.)

(Modified schedule for July only)

**Wednesday, July 20**

| Time | Activity | Location |
|---|---|---|
| 7:30–8:30 A.M. | Meet with unit manager, palliative care/rehab Palliative Care | Manager's Office |
| 8:30–9:30 A.M. | Meet with unit manager | 7 East Oncology Manager's Office |
| 9:30 – 10:30 A.M. | Meet with unit manager | 7 West Mgr.-Office—7 West |
| 10:30–11:00 A.M. | Catch-up/emails | |
| 11:00–12:00 P.M. | Lunch | |
| 12:00–3:15 P.M. | Teletracking/Med Rec/Optilink | Annex 4 Classroom |
| 3:15–4:00 P.M. | Independent time | |

**Thursday, July 21**

| Time | Activity | Location |
|---|---|---|
| 7:30–4:00 P.M. | Med-surg curriculum—day 2 (Modified schedule for July only) | Classroom D |

**Friday, July 22**

| Time | Activity | Location |
|---|---|---|
| 8:00–10:00 A.M. | Attend debriefing class | Sim Lab |
| 10:00–11:00 A.M. | Meet with AHA training center coordinator ACLS, BLS | TCC office |
| 11:00–12:00 P.M. | Lunch | |
| 12:00 –4:30 P.M. | Independent time to work on individual needs | |

---

### Exhibit 9.1 | Sample Orientation Schedule for New Medical/Surgical Educator (cont.)

*Source: Summa Health System. Used with permission.*

**Other experiences to be arranged in the future:**

- Observe preparation/welcome for NEONI students
- Educational Leadership Meeting
- RN Preceptor Workshop
- Other experiences as needed

---

# References

American Nurses Association and National Nursing Staff Development Organization. (2010). *Nursing professional development: Scope and standards of practice.* Silver Spring MD: Nursesbook.org.

Avillion, A.E., & Buchwald, D. (2010). *Nursing orientation program builder: Tools for a successful new hire program.* Danvers, MA: HCPro.

Bruce, S.L. (ed). (2013). *Core curriculum for nursing professional development.* (4th ed). Chicago, IL: Association for Nursing Professional Development.

Summa Health System. (2012). Orientation Schedule for Medical/Surgical Director.

# Chapter 10

# Performance Appraisals, Peer Review, and Professional Development Plans

## Learning Objective

**After reading this chapter, the participant should be able to:**

☑ Create a development plan based on performance appraisal and peer review feedback

## Using the Checklist for Yearly Performance Appraisals

Educators can use the performance criteria in the tool as documentation that they have achieved expected competencies for yearly performance appraisals. Administrators can use the criteria when evaluating the performance of their staff members. Typically, performance appraisals are based on the competencies included in the position description, and if the position description uses the competencies in this tool, then the performance appraisal can easily flow from the position description.

Since the criteria are all measurable, the tool provides an objective assessment of staff competence. Both administrators and educators can use the tool to identify goals for professional growth for the next appraisal period.

Some organizations require documentation of achievement of selected competencies as part of the performance appraisal process. The expectations vary based on roles and responsibilities and a sample of a competency checklist developed specifically from this tool is provided in exhibit 10.1. Another example of an equipment-related competency is provided in exhibit 10.2.

## Exhibit 10.1| Sample Competency Checklist

### ANYTOWN HEALTH SYSTEM
### DEPARTMENT OF EDUCATION
### ANNUAL COMPETENCY PERFORMANCE
### QUALITY OF INSTRUCTION

NAME: _____ Title: _____ Unit: _____

| CRITICAL ELEMENTS | MET | NOT MET | COMMENTS |
|---|---|---|---|
| Develops objectives that are relevant, realistic, and measurable. | | | |
| Incorporates teaching/learning strategies to address identified needs and goals. | | | |
| Uses up-to-date and accurate resources/materials in presentation. | | | |
| Picks up on verbal and nonverbal cues during session. | | | |
| Ensures any handouts are easily read, free of errors, and attractively designed. | | | |
| Bases audiovisuals on the size of the group, setting, and equipment available. | | | |
| Provides pertinent information useful to practice. | | | |

Reference: Brunt, B.A. (2007). *Competencies for Staff Educators: Tools to Evaluate and Enhance Nursing Professional Development*. Marblehead, MA: HCPro.

☐ Passed                    ☐ Needs to Repeat

Validated by: _____ Date:_____

Original Date: _____

Reviewed: _____

Revised: _____

*Source: Summa Health System. (2013). Quality of instruction checklist. Reprinted with permission.*

Exhibit 10.2 | Sample Equipment-Related Competency

## ANYTOWN HEALTH SYSTEM

## DEPARTMENT OF EDUCATION

## Use of AED for BLS Instructor

## Competency Checklist

Name: _____ Title: _____ Unit: _____

| CRITICAL ELEMENTS | MET | NOT MET | COMMENTS |
|---|---|---|---|
| Reviews steps of AED algorithm:<br>    a. Assesses patient and establishes unresponsiveness | | | |
|     b. Calls for EMS/defibrillator/Code Blue | | | |
|     c. Starts CPR | | | |
| Turns AED on. | | | |
| Attaches AED with correct size pads to bare chest:<br>Below right clavicle to right of sternum (upper right of chest to right of breastbone, below collarbone) | | | |
| Left midaxillary line at level of 5th intercostal space (left of nipple, a few inches below armpit) | | | |
| Initiates analysis, after clearing the victim. | | | |
| Clears the victim and delivers shock as appropriate. | | | |
| Continues CPR for two full minutes beginning with chest compressions. | | | |
| Reassesses with AED, repeating steps 4 and 5. | | | |

☐ **Passed**      ☐ **Needs to Repeat**

Validated by: _____ Date: _____
                (Name and Title)

**Reference:** BLS for Healthcare Providers, 2010, American Heart Association.

**Reviewed:** ____
**Revised:** ____

*Source: Summa Health System. (2011). Use of ALD for BLS instructor competency checklist. Reprinted with permission.*

Since performance appraisal forms vary from institution to institution, a sample evaluation form is not included in this chapter. However, information from the competencies on the checklist can be used as a guide in determining whether individuals met the competencies included on the performance appraisal.

# Peer Review

Peer review is becoming increasingly important in relation to quality care and standards of practice. One of the standards in the scope and standards for nursing professional development (NPD) on professional practice evaluation states "the nursing professional development specialist evaluates his or her own practice in relation to professional practice standards and guidelines, and relevant statutes, rules, and regulations," and one of the measurement criteria is "participates in peer review" (American Nurses Association [ANA] & National Nursing Staff Development Organization [NNSDO], 2010, p. 34).

Peer review is the evaluation of an individual nurse's professional performance by another nurse, or evaluation by one's peers (Harrington & Smith, 2010). Peer review allows an educator's actions to be evaluated by someone practicing as an educator with the goal of identifying opportunities to improve practice. Peer review data are often used as part of the performance evaluation process.

Systematic peer review is needed to ensure the quality and competency of the professional through collaboration, communication, and accountability. Contemporary peer review principles include the following:

- Peer review involves the use of established standards for the evaluation of a nurse's practice using the following evidence-based peer review principles:
  - A peer is someone of the same rank.
  - Peer review is practice-focused.
  - Feedback is timely, routine, and a continuous expectation.
  - Peer review fosters a continuous learning culture of patient safety and best practice.
  - Feedback is not anonymous.
  - Feedback incorporates the developmental stage of the nurse (George & Haig-Haitman, 2012, pp. 27–28).

# Professional Development Plan

An NPD specialist can also use this tool to create a professional development plan. Since the tool is a comprehensive description of the full range of novice-to-expert staff development practice, it is not anticipated that many educators will meet all the competencies. Individual educators can use this tool to identify areas for growth and the performance criteria can provide a road map of steps to take to meet a particular competency. This will provide a systematic method to plan for ongoing growth and development in a particular role.

For example, if an NPD specialist has never written a grant application and wants to write one, he or she can look at the performance criteria under that competency to determine how to proceed. Steps in the process include, but are not limited to, the following:

- Identifying potential sources of funding

- Seeking assistance from an experienced grant writer

- Determining a budget and associated expenses for the project

- Assisting with or completing a grant proposal according to guidelines

- Describing other funding sources/how the project will continue after funding expires

- Writing or assisting with writing the report of findings to the funding agency

The development plan should include the experiences needed to gain the required skills, as well as specific timelines to achieve those.

TIP: Including specific deadlines can help avoid procrastination.

# Reflect on Development

Critical reflection is an important aspect of creating a professional development plan. Educators need to contemplate and reflect on their past experiences as they develop a plan. Identify areas of strength, as well as areas that may require further development. Critically analyzing specific situations that occurred can be helpful in identifying different ways of dealing with a similar situation if it occurs again.

Some of the qualities that enable reflection include:

- Having an open mind

- Being responsible

- Considering all sides of the situation

- Considering outcomes of actions

- Taking active control of one's own education, development, and practice

Using a professional development plan provides a road map for future learning opportunities and professional growth.

This chapter reviewed how the NPD competency tool can be used in performance appraisals, peer review, and professional development.

# References

American Nurses Association and National Nursing Staff Development Organization. (2010). *Nursing professional development: Scope and standards of practice.* Silver Spring, MD: Nursesbook.org.

Brunt, B.A. (2007). *Competencies for staff educators: Tools to evaluate and enhance nursing professional development.* Danvers, MA: HCPro.

George, V., & Haag-Heitman, B. (2012). Differentiating peer review and the annual performance review. *Nurse Leader,* 10(1), 26–28. doi: 10.1016/j.mnl/2011.11.005.

Harrington, L.C., & Smith, M. (2008). *Nursing peer review: A practical approach to promoting professional nursing accountability.* Danvers, MA: HCPro.

Summa Health System (2011). *Use of AED for BLS Instructors Competency Checklist.* Akron, OH: Summa Health System.

Summa Health System (2013). *Quality of Instruction Competency Checklist.* Akron, OH: Summa Health System.

# Chapter 11

# Creating a Professional Portfolio

The following definition of portfolio from the 2000 ANA standards, which was included as an appendix in the new standards (American Nurses Association [ANA] & National Nursing Staff Development Organization [NNSDO], 2010), is presented to guide the discussion in this chapter:

**Portfolio:** Material documenting the professional development, career planning, demonstration of learning, and maintenance of continuing professional nursing competence of the individual nurse.

## Why Create a Portfolio?

One of the standards of professional performance for nursing professional development (NPD) is that the NPD specialist maintains current knowledge and competency in nursing and professional development practice. There are also standards relating to enhancing quality and effectiveness of NPD practice, as well as evaluation of one's own practice. A professional portfolio is one way to document ongoing, continuing professional nursing competence. NPD specialists need to develop a personal portfolio, in addition to helping nurses and other staff members develop their own portfolios.

Although portfolios are not widely utilized in the United States, this author believes they will become more prevalent in the future. Since 1995, the United Kingdom Central Council for Nursing, Midwifery and Health Visiting (UKCC) has required individuals on the professional register to use a

Personal Professional Profile, which is like a portfolio. A personal portfolio is a private collection of evidence that demonstrates the continuing acquisition of skills, knowledge, attitudes, understanding, and achievement. It is both retrospective and prospective, as well as reflecting the current stage of development of the individual. Portfolios enable individuals to keep a record of their personal and professional development, professional experiences, and qualifications.

Portfolios may include the following components:

- Professional credentials

- Continuing education

- Leadership activities

- Narrative self-reflection of practice

- Documentation of the relevance of professional learning experiences

- Examples demonstrating competence in a certain area

Creating a profile is an excellent opportunity for individuals to take stock of their life and career in the context of their future educational and work-related activities. Although some people may have already given a great deal of thought to their future career options, many have not spent time focusing on the direction they would like to take. It is worth investing time in reviewing one's situation to ensure that choices are genuine, realistic, and achievable.

> Tip: Taking the time to develop a portfolio is a great way to invest in oneself and one's career.

When making decisions about future career options, individuals need to think about personal values and interests they need to satisfy in order to be fulfilled and happy in what they chose to do. Values affect how individuals communicate with others and have a strong influence on personal and professional decisions. Professional values to consider are listed in Figure 11.1.

Figure 11.1 | Professional values to consider

| Promotion | Money |
|---|---|
| Working conditions | Hours |
| Helping others | Relationships |
| Recognition | Learning |
| Security | Time |
| Stress-free work | Diversity |
| Freedom | Admiration |
| Manager | Practitioner |
| Other values that are important | |

# Types of Portfolios

Andre (2010) identified three basic approaches/types of portfolios, which are:

1. Learning portfolio—used to direct, document, and make explicit the learning process

2. Credentialing portfolio—used to present an argument of competence that is durable over time and to different circumstances

3. Showcase portfolio—used to display completed works that may not necessarily be accompanied by reflective text or justification

The primary purpose will determine the format and approach used for each portfolio.

## E-portfolios

E-portfolios are defined as an electronic platform used to structure, store, and retrieve information, including text, graphic, and audio and video materials. Andre (2010) suggested that the use of e-portfolios by professionals is likely to become mainstream practice in the next few years.

This was verified by Green, Wyllie, and Jackson (2014), who did a review of the literature on electronic portfolios in nursing education. They found that e-portfolios facilitated accountability and autonomy because they encourage students to take responsibility for their learning needs, as well as the direction, progress, and quality of that learning. In addition, they found them to have a major advantage over traditional portfolios due to their portability and adaptability, as the text and artifacts are able to be held in a central repository where they can be assembled electronically and manipulated and reversioned to suit differing audiences.

# Building a Portfolio

The actual construction and organization of a portfolio varies depending on the individual and the organization's requirements. A general guide to constructing the portfolio includes the following information:

- Introduction
- Details of professional experience, knowledge, and skills
- Demonstration of achievement of required competencies
- Testimonials, references, or samples of work

Developing a portfolio provides individuals with the opportunity to be creative and include materials unique to them. Examples could include reports, research data, educational programs designed, lesson plans, and other material, as well as photographs, articles, poems, or short stories.

Tips: When building a portfolio:

- Be selective: Include only relevant material
- Be clear and concise: Make it easy to read and understand
- Be coherent: Have each section flow logically from the previous section
- Be professional: Consider the presentation—it should be typed and grammatically correct and have the same style throughout

NPD specialists can use this tool to generate ideas on how to document achievement of a particular competency. They can also use it as a means of identifying areas for development, using strategies such as reflective practice and critical incident analysis. The professional portfolio can provide a vehicle for communicating competence, professional development, and skills that could be transferable to another area.

# Helping Others Develop Professional Portfolios

In addition to developing their own personal portfolio, educators may be asked to assist others in developing a portfolio. In this role, the NPD specialist will be helping the individual make sense of the knowledge and skills he or she already has and make decisions about what should be included in the portfolio. This facilitation would involve the following skills:

- Enabling: Supporting individuals through the development of their portfolio. This would include active listening skills and creating an environment in which individuals are able to speak openly and in confidence about their thoughts and feelings.

- Educational counseling: Helping individuals discover, clarify, assess, and understand their learning in order to plan realistic current and future educational aims and career goals.

- Advising: Helping individuals interpret information and make decisions based on their planned learning needs.

- Assessing: Assisting individuals to develop confidence in self-assessment and to evaluate the scope of their learning. Through self-assessment individuals will be much more likely to take control of the profile, to make informed choices about what it should include, and to have ownership of it.

- Informing: Providing information about learning opportunities and professional development policies.

Questions to ask the individual developing the portfolio include:

1. Why are you developing a portfolio?
2. What do you know about the process of developing a portfolio?
3. When do you need/want the portfolio to be completed?
4. What type of portfolio do you want?
5. What skills do you already have to complete it?

6. What skills do you need to develop?

7. How would you like me to help you with this process?

8. What help can you expect from others?

Establish an action plan with timelines and ground rules to ensure completion of the portfolio within the desired time frame.

## Use of Portfolios in Education

Garrett, MacPhee, and Jackson (2013) completed an action-research study to evaluate the implementation of an electronic portfolio tool for the assessment of clinical competence in a bachelor of science in nursing program. The study included instructor and student surveys and focus groups, as well as website tracking analytics and descriptive statistics to explore trends in e-portfolio usage. Instructors valued the convenience of the e-portfolios, improved transparency, improved ability to track student progress, and enhanced theory-practice links and the competency-based assessment framework. Students valued accessibility and convenience but expressed concerns over assessment date openness and processes for standardization.

McColgan and Blackwood (2009) completed a systematic review protocol on the use of teaching portfolios for educators. A teaching portfolio is an educator's personal collection of factual accomplishments and strengths in teaching. It portrays the quality and scope of an individual's teaching performance and is commonly categorized into three parts:

1. Personal material, such as personal reflections and statements of teaching responsibilities

2. Material from others, such as peer and students evaluation

3. Products of teaching and student learning

The teaching portfolio has been identified as a professional development tool that provides a method of linking self-development with enhanced teaching and learning practices. Some colleges have implemented a teaching portfolio as a method to judge teaching performance for promotion and tenure.

This chapter described portfolios, including the various types. It provided suggestions for building a portfolio and helping others develop portfolios. It also outlined how portfolios are used in education.

# References

Andre, K. (2010), E-portfolios for the aspiring professional. *Collegian,* 17, 119–124. doi: 10.1016/j.colegn.2009.10.005.

American Nurses Association and National Nursing Staff Development Organization. (2010). *Nursing professional development: Scope and standards of practice.* Silver Spring, MD: Nursesbook.org.

Garrett, B.M., MacPhee, M., & Jackson, C. (2013). Evaluation of an eportfolio for the assessment of clinical competence in a baccalaureate nursing program. *Nurse Education Today,* 33, 1207–1213. doi: 10.1016/j.nedt.2012.06.015.

Green, J., Wyllie, A., & Jackson, D. (2014). Electronic portfolios in nursing education: A review of the literature. *Nurse Education in Practice,* 14, 4–8. *http://dx.doi.org/10.1016/j.nepr.2013.08.011.*

McColgan, K., & Blackwood, B. (2009). A systematic review protocol on the use of teaching portfolios for educators in further and higher education. *Journal of Advanced Nursing,* 65(12), 2500–2507. doi: 10.1111/j.1365-2648.2009.05189.x.

# Chapter 12

# Developing Cultural Competence

| Learning Objective |
| --- |
| **After reading this chapter, the participant should be able to:** |
| ☑ Discuss the importance of cultural competence in the educational role |

The following definitions of key concepts are presented to guide the discussion.

**Culturally competent care:** Care that adapts interventions to the cultural needs and preferences (ethnic and religious beliefs, values, and practices) of diverse patients.

**Cultural competence:** An ongoing process in which the healthcare provider continuously strives to effectively work within the cultural context of the client. This includes the integration of cultural awareness, cultural desire, cultural knowledge, cultural skills, and cultural encounters.

## Cultural Competence and Nursing Professional Development Specialists

There are several core competencies outlined in the new standards for nursing professional development (NPD) American Nurses Association [ANA] & National Nursing Staff Development Organization [NNSDO], 2010) that relate to cultural competence: "implements a variety of teaching strategies tailored to the learners' characteristics, learning needs, cultural perspectives, and outcome objectives" and "plans NPD programs that are culturally relevant and that incorporate concepts of multicultural and multigenerational education" (p. 14).

The National Culturally and Linguistically Appropriate Services (CLAS) Standards in Health and Health Care intend to advance health equity, improve quality, and help eliminate healthcare disparities by establishing a blueprint for health and healthcare organizations to provide culturally and linguistically appropriate service delivery that meets the healthcare needs of the population served.

Diallo and McGrath (2013) noted that 2012 census data stated that Asians and Hispanics are the fastest-growing ethnic groups in the U.S. population. Therefore, the majority of patients receiving primary and preventive care under the changes with the Accountable Care Act will be among today's minority groups. So, more than ever before, time needs to be spent on analysis and discussion of how these changes will shape the quality of care to be culturally sensitive.

Cultural competence builds first on an awareness of one's own cultural perspective and then adds knowledge about the perspective of another culture on the same issue. Since NPD specialists teach learners who represent a variety of cultures, they need to consider the affect culture has on learning (Garbutt, 2013.

The first step to ensuring cultural competence is a cultural assessment, which includes the following:

- Identification of learner's cultural understanding and norms
- Identification of learner beliefs, values, and practices that could assist or interfere with learning
- Awareness of the educator to better understand the learners' frame of reference

Too often health professionals form their own cultural perspectives, fail to modify their approaches to be responsive to the needs of culturally diverse learners, and fail to recognize the ineffectiveness of their teaching. Many nurses identify a lack of knowledge, skills, and confidence to care for patients from diverse backgrounds, and cultural content in many nursing school curriculums is limited.

Studies have demonstrated the positive impact of training in improving the cultural competence of healthcare providers. Training has been shown to improve communication across cultural and linguistic differences, as well as to increase knowledge and self-efficacy.

# Barriers to Cultural Competence

Barriers to cultural competence are outlined in Figure 12.1.

Figure 12.1 | Barriers to Cultural Competence

| |
|---|
| Lack of awareness of differences |
| Lack of time |
| Ethnocentrism, bias, and prejudice |
| Lack of skills to address differences |
| Lack of organizational support |

# Strategies to Promote Cultural Competence

NPD specialists can play a key role in improving cultural competence both in the initial orientation program as well as in ongoing staff education. Suggested topics to include in education are the relevance of cultural competence, culture and health culture, intercultural communication, language issues, and skills application. Avillion (2012) described cultural issues to incorporate into education about cultural diversity. Among these were eye contact, handshake, personal space, dress, business etiquette, response to pain, dietary issues, family spokesperson issues, caring for persons of the opposite sex, facial expressions and gestures, and body language.

Many schools of nursing have implemented strategies to recruit, retain, and prepare a workforce that is more representative of the country's demographics. In addition, many organizations are also exploring how to achieve a more diverse workforce to provide culturally competent care.

Lack of awareness for both educators and staff can be overcome with information and resources about different cultures and using speakers from various ethnic groups. Lack of time can be overcome by changing the healthcare providers' mind-set and encouraging them to put themselves in patients' shoes, thereby allowing them to identify potential needs.

Ethnocentrism is the belief in the superiority of one's own ethnic group, which can lead to bias and prejudice against individuals who are not of the same ethnic group. Focusing on intercultural communication skills can help combat this problem, as can teaching skills to address differences, which can be part of the overall awareness campaign.

Many staff members are not aware of the cultural diversity resources available. Most organizations have a number of resources available on cultural competence, including policies and procedures, resource materials, individuals with expertise in that area, and language-interpreting services.

NPD specialists can document cultural competence by preparing and presenting information for staff on this topic or by describing a situation where they addressed cultural competence in an educational program.

Bourque Bearskin (2011) summed up the components of culturally respectful practice in the following ways:

R—Reflect deeply on your own cultural values and beliefs

E—Examine and question assumptions and biases in practice

S—Share and recognize ethical space of nurse-patient relationships

P—Participate and celebrate cultural uniqueness

E—Engage in relationship building

C—Create open and trusting environments

T—Treat people with dignity and compassion (p. 557)

## Research

Educational programs can make a difference in achieving cultural competence. Hawala-Druy and Hill (2012) conducted a research study on the effectiveness of a semester-long university course that promoted positive and culturally competent outcomes for culturally diverse and largely millennial students. Students were from various health professions, including nursing, pharmacy, and allied health sciences. This was a qualitative and quantitative study, which measured students' level of cultural awareness, competence, and proficiency pre- and post-educational intervention. There were statistically significant changes in the mean scores pre- and post-test. Student feedback was that they liked the eclectic, creative, evidence-based interdisciplinary activities and culturally congruent teaching strategies used in this course.

This chapter defined cultural competence and described implications for the NPD specialist. Barriers to cultural competence and strategies to promote cultural competence were outlined.

# References

American Nurses Association and National Nursing Staff Development Organization (2010). *Nursing professional development: Scope and standards of practice.* Silver Spring, MD: Nursesbook.org.

Avillion, A.E. (2012). *The path to stress-free nursing professional development: 50 no-nonsense solutions to everyday challenges.* Danvers, MA: HCPro.

Bourque Bearskin, R.L. (2011). A critical lens on culture in nursing practice. *Nursing Ethics,* 18, 548–549. doi: 10/1177/0969733011408048.

Diallo, A.F., & McGrath, J.M. (2013). A glance at the future of cultural competency in healthcare. *Newborn and Infant Nursing Reviews,* 13, 121–123. doi:10.1053/j.nainr.2013.07.003.

Garbutt, S.J. (2013). Cultural diversity awareness: Implications for the nursing professional development specialist. In S.L. Bruce (ed.), *Core curriculum for nursing professional development* (4th ed, p 107–117). Chicago, IL: Association for Nursing Professional Development.

Hawala-Druy, S., & Hill, M.H. (2012). Interdisciplinary: Cultural competency and culturally congruent education for millennials in health professions. *Nurse Education Today,* 32, 772–778. doi: 10.1016/j. nedt.2012.05.002.

National standards on culturally and linguistically appropriate services (CLAS). (n.d.). Retrieved from *http:// minorityhealth.hhs.gov/templates/browse.aspx?lvl = 2&lvllD = 15.*

# Chapter 13

# Understanding Generational Differences

## Characteristics of the Various Generations

There is some variation among authors on the specific time frames and influences for each generation. The years most commonly cited in the literature are used here. The most variation is in Generation Y and Generation Z; some authors list four generations and have Generation Y as being born between 1981 and 2002. Many different terms are used for Generation Y: millennials, nexters, gen net, and linked generation.

There are five generations described in this chapter:

1. Traditionalists—born between 1926 and 1945

2. Baby Boomers—born between 1946 and 1964

3. Generation X—born between 1965 and 1980

4. Generation Y—born between 1981 and 1994

5. Generation Z—born between 1994 and 2004

Each generation has unique communication styles, motivators, values, expectations, and career goals. It should be understood that not all individuals who fall into one generation are alike, and we need to be careful not to label or stereotype people. Lower (2006) noted the way people typically fulfill the characteristics of each generation can be demonstrated by a bell-shaped curve. Most results will be in the middle, while those at either end will be one or two standard deviations from the norm. Some people will be almost completely unlike the characteristics ascribed to a particular generation, while other will be almost 100% like the description.

## Traditionalists

Also known as Veterans or the Silent Generations, Traditionalists were influenced by World War II and the Great Depression. The political and economic uncertainty of these times created a generation generally considered to be financially conservative, hardworking, and cautious.

Characteristics of Traditionalists include a strong work ethic, loyalty, respect for authority, adherence to rules, and consistency. They prefer to communicate through phone calls, one-on-one meetings, or written communication.

## Baby Boomers

Baby Boomers, the largest group in the workplace, were influenced by the hippie movement, the Vietnam War, the ideals of John F. Kennedy and Martin Luther King, Jr., the Civil Rights movement, and a healthy postwar economy. Characteristics of Baby Boomers include being workaholics, questioning authority, and valuing individualism. They are idealistic, confident, and good decision-makers and have a sense of entitlement. They spend freely to keep up with the Joneses, and many are not financially prepared for retirement. They prefer to communicate by phone or in person.

## Generation X

Once the Traditionalists retire, this will be the smallest group in the workforce. Generation Xers were influenced by dual-career households, latchkey kids, increased divorce rates, the Challenger disaster, Google, Amazon, and technological advances. Generation X views work as a challenge; they like some structure or direction but view themselves as self-reliant. Cynical and pessimistic, they are rarely loyal to an organization, as they seek balance between work, family, and leisure. They are tech savvy but often lack basic social skills. They prefer to communicate via phones and other electronic devices.

## Generation Y

Generation Y was influenced by advances in technology, the nation's uncertainly after 9/11, the Clinton scandal, and public acts of violence. Generation Y would like work to be more fun, and many would like to work from home. They consider work a means to an end, are multitaskers, have a sense of entrepreneurialism, are goal oriented, and value teamwork.

They typically have respect and affection for their parents, volunteer readily, and welcome guidance. They prefer to communicate using technology, such as cell phones, texting/instant messaging, and email.

## Generation Z

Sometimes referred to as the iGeneration, in regard to the technologies popular with this group (e.g., iTunes, iPhones), Generation Z is a highly connected generation that has never known a time without computers or cell phones. Generation Z was influenced by disasters such as Hurricane Katrina, the earthquake in Haiti, and the recession of 2008. They are close to family, confident, and open to change. They have a sense of civic duty, sociability, morality, diversity, and street smarts. They too prefer to communicate using technology.

# Teaching Strategies with the Various Generations

There has been a fair amount published on suggested teaching styles with the various generations (Avillion, 2012; Avillion & Buchwald, 2010; Bell, 2013; Engvall, 2013), and the information below summarizes that information.

Traditionalists:

- Make sure learning objectives are clearly stated and understood
- Provide resources for help with distance learning if using unfamiliar technology
- Acknowledge life experiences
- Avoid small print on handouts—nothing less than 12-point font
- Motivate them by explaining how education will improve job performance
- Allow them to practice skills before demonstrating them in front of a group
- Provide lots of opportunities for feedback
- Create an organized learning environment

Baby Boomers
- Use icebreakers and team-building activities
- Avoid role-playing activities
- Offer resources that pertain to their roles and responsibilities
- Assume the role of a facilitator rather than a rigid authority figure
- Explain how learning activities will enhance job performance
- Allow them to practice skills before demonstrating them in front of a group
- Provide a structured environment and clear guidelines

Generation X
- Offer as many self-directed activities as possible
- Use hands-on learning and role play
- Allow plenty of time for discussion and questions

- Provide visual stimulation, such as pictures, graphs, and tables
- Use technology in programs
- Make yourself available to listen to questions and concerns

Generation Y

- Use blended learning that is convenient and flexible
- Encourage participation in mentoring programs
- Incorporate music and games in education
- Provide opportunities for personal interaction with learning
- Offer lists of reading resources
- Offer education on-demand and at times convenient to them
- Teach through active experimentation and seeing concepts in action

Generation Z

- Provide flexible, on-demand education
- Incorporate simulation experiences
- Incorporate fun as a part of learning
- Keep programs up to date and current
- Be prepared for multitasking in the classroom setting
- Focus on how to access, synthesize, and integrate information

Riggs (2013a, 2013b) discussed the application of different communication and interaction techniques to improve the efficiency of communication with a nursing workforce with multiple generations. She provided two sample scenarios, one demonstrating excellent communication and one demonstrating a need for improved communication. Knowledge of generational differences, characteristics, and work habits will enable employees to collaborate efficiently with each other in the workplace.

Gallo (2011) outlined the best method of education to use with the various generations. See Figure 13-1.

## Figure 13.1 | Best Method of Education

| Generation | Learning style | Self-directed/ self-learning modules | Traditional classroom instruction | Case presentations | Role playing | Online education | Online education with synchronous and asynchronous activities | Webinar | Simulation with debriefing |
|---|---|---|---|---|---|---|---|---|---|
| **Veteran** | Traditional classroom orientation Face-to-face or written communication | X | X | X | X | X | | | |
| **Baby boomer** | Direct, personal, face-to-face communication and group participation Comfortable with the use of computers | X | X | X | X | X | X | X | X |
| **Generation X** | High-tech videos or computer-aided instruction Entertaining fast paced information with problem solving opportunities | X | | X | X | X | X | X | X |
| **Generation Y** | Technological and computer preference | X | | X | X | X | X | X | X |

Reprinted from "Beyond the classroom using technology to meet the educational needs of multigenerational perinatal nurses." By Ana-Maria Gallo (2011). *The Journal of Perinatal & Neonatal Nursing, 25*(2), p. 198. Copyright 2011 by Lippincott, Williams & Wilkins Inc. Reprinted with permission.

## Strategies for Managers

Generational differences present challenges to contemporary nurse managers working in a healthcare environment that is complex and dynamic in terms of managing nurses who think and behave in a different way because of differing personal and generational values, especially in the three Cs of communication, commitment, and compensation. Hendricks and Cope (2012) provided suggestions for dealing with this.

Nurse managers who recognize and value each generation's approach to communication are instrumental in creating a cohesive workplace. Ground rules should reinforce the importance of respect and tolerance for all generations. Highlighting mutual team goals and keeping patient care as the focal point will promote effective work. In addition to face-to-face or written communication, managers must also include technology.

A work environment where nurses' differences are considered is central to building commitment. If the nurse manager develops an appreciation for the ways generations value work and the balance of work in their lives, it helps to create an environment where individuals, as representatives of a cohort, feel valued. This subsequently builds strategies for retaining staff and promoting satisfaction in the workplace

Knowledge of generational staff mix allows the nurse manager to develop a work environment that manages individuals in a way that best suits their motivational characteristics. Managers can vary the reward system for each generational cohort. For instance, if boomers are motivated by money and the two younger groups by time off, the manager can offer each group what it wants most or provide a generation-specific reward.

Lower (2006) provided a variety of practical tips for managing the multigenerational workforce in the area of schedules, work-life balance, learning, involvement on the unit, performance reviews, feedback and promotion, working together, and retention and recognition.

## Research

Rainmaker Thinking has done extensive research on generational differences (Tulgan, 2003). The results of their first 10-year study from 1993 to 2003 identified six key findings:

1. Work has become more demanding on employees.
2. Employer-employee relationships have become less hierarchical and more transactional.
3. Employers are moving away from long-term employment relationships.
4. Employees have less confidence in long-term rewards and greater expectations for short-term rewards.
5. Immediate supervisors are now the most important people in the workplace.
6. Supervising employees now requires more time and skill on the part of managers.

Their research continued from 2003 to 2013 (Rainmaker Thinking, 2013b). During this time they conducted one-on-one interviews with 6,098 managers and 3,177 nonmanagers from 362 different organizations and also conducted 407 in-person focus groups. In addition, they collected narrative responses to open-ended question from 37,419 managers and 61,797 nonmanagers from 891 different organizations. Specific tactics that were identified to bring out the best in the Generation X and Generation Z employees included:

1. Get them onboard fast with the right messages.

2. Get them up to speed quickly and turn them into knowledge workers.

3. Give them the gift of context.

4. Teach them to care about delivering great customer services.

5. Teach them how to manage themselves.

6. Teach them how to be managed by you.

7. Retain the best of them, one day at a time (Rainmaker Thinking, 2013a).

Robinson and colleagues (2012) conducted a research study on generational differences and learning style preferences. Results from the 122 nurses who completed the study indicated a combination of years in practice, time lapsed since last educational program ended, current school enrollment, degree earned, and generation-influenced preferred learning style. Results indicated the divergent and accommodator learning styles were more likely to be preferred by those from older generations and by those who have more time lapsed since they finished their educational program. Conversely, assimilator and converger learning styles may be preferred by those who have fewer years of practice, recently completed their nursing program, and/or are currently enrolled in an educational program, have completed an advanced degree, and are from a younger generation.

This chapter provided information on the various generations, including teaching strategies that are most effective with each group. Strategies for managers to deal with a multigenerational workforce were outlined, as well as some current research in this area.

# References

Avillion, A.E. (2012). *The path to stress-free nursing professional development: 50 no-nonsense solutions to everyday challenges.* Danvers, MA: HCPro.

Avillion, A.E., & Buchwach, D. (2010). *Nursing orientation program builder: Tools for a successful new hire program.* Marblehead, MA: HCPro.

Bell, J.A. (2013). Five generations in the nursing workforce: Implications for nursing professional development. *Journal for Nurses in Staff Development*, 29(4), 205–210. doi: 10.1097/NND.0b013e31829aedd4.

Engvall, J.C. (2013). Generational differences. In S.L. Bruce, (ed.), *Core curriculum for nursing professional development* (4th ed, pp.89–105), Chicago, IL: Association for Nursing Professional Development.

Hendricks, J.M., & Cope, V.C. (2012). Generational diversity: What nurse managers need to know. *Journal of Advanced Nursing*, 69(3), 717–725. doi: 10.1111/j.1365-2648.2012.06079.x.

Lower, J.S. (2006). *A practical guide to managing the multigenerational workforce: Skill for nurse managers.* Marblehead, MA: HCPro.

Gallo, A. (2011). Beyond the classroom using technology to meet the educational needs of multigenerational perinatal nurses. *Journal of Perinatal and Neonatal Nursing*, 25(2), 19, 195-19. doi: 10.1097/JPN.0b013e3182163993.

Rainmaker Thinking (2013a). *Bringing out the best in young talent: Managing generations Y & Z.* Retrieved from *http://rainmakerthinking.com/assets/uploads/2013/10/Bringing-Out-the-Best-in-Young-Talent.pdf.*

Rainmaker Thinking (2013b). *The research: Our ten year workplace study—2003–2013.* Retrieved from *http://rainmakerthinking.com/assets/uploads/2013/10.Generational-SHift.pdf.*

Riggs, C.L. (2013a). Multiple generations in the nursing workplace: Part I. *The Journal of Continuing Education in Nursing*, 44(3), 105–106. doi: 10.3928/00220124-20130222-04.

Riggs, C.L. (2013b). Multiple generations in the nursing workplace: Part II. *The Journal of Continuing Education in Nursing*, 44(4), 153–154. doi: 10.3928/00220124-20130327-19.

Robinson, J., Scollan-Koliopoulos, M., Kamienski, M., & Burke, K. (2012). Generational differences and learning style preferences in nurses from a large metropolitan medical center. *Journal for Nurses in Staff Development*, 28(4), 166–172. doi: 10.1097/NND.0b013e31825dfae5.

Tulgan, B. (2003). *Generational shift: What we saw at the workplace revolution. Executive Summary: Key finding of our ten year workplace study* (1993–2003). New Haven, CT: Rainmaker Thinking Inc.

# Chapter 14

# Applications of the Competencies

*By Julia W. Aucoin, DNS, RN-BC, CNE*

This chapter focuses on suggested applications of the competencies. Some are logical and some are provocative so that new and creative uses will be considered. Each will describe what is needed to make the application work.

## Graduate Nursing Education Programs

There is continued value to graduate nursing education programs that focus on both the academic nurse educator and the nursing professional development (NPD) roles. Content should be evidence-based, as are these competencies. A balanced approach must be used when presenting both roles, and thus when presenting the competencies of academic educators they can be compared and contrasted to those of the NPD specialist.

Educators can create exercises where learners self-assess, discuss the applicability of each competency to the other's role, create a competency checklist to use in the graduate practicum, or write a development plan for all or a portion of the listed competencies. This will allow the competencies to be developed, embraced, and employed when learners enter the practice setting. The graduate course in professional development can be organized around the competencies to be sure that essential content is covered and course objectives are appropriate to the role. It is necessary, then, that the graduate nursing education program recognizes the validity of both the academic and practice roles and presents them with similar evidence.

## Scope and Standards of Nursing Professional Development

*Nursing Professional Development: Scope and Standards of Practice* was last published in 2010 (American Nurses Association and National Nursing Staff Development Organization). The revision resulted in clarity around the current responsibilities of the nursing professional development (NPD) specialist—career development, education leadership, program management, and compliance—reflecting core competencies. The roles have been clarified to reflect and describe fully the scope of practice, embedded in the standards. The revised roles of educator/facilitator, educator/academic liaison, change agent/team member, researcher/consultant, leader communicator, and collaborator/advisor/member continue to evolve as NPD evidence continues to grow. To differentiate the practice of the NPD specialist from the academic educator it is essential to draw attention to the National League for Nursing (NLN, 2012). *The Scope of Practice for Academic Nurse Educators* fully addresses the academic competencies (NLN, 2007) for this complementary role. This delineation between the scope of the roles was considered carefully by the content expert panel who developed the revised *Nursing Professional Development: Scope and Standards of Practice.*

## Resource for Certification Exam

These competencies should be used as a resource for the NPD certification exam prepared by the American Nurses Credentialing Center (ANCC). The content expert panel should include them as a reference for item development and study materials. In addition, the test plan should be examined to be sure that it reflects the competencies. When a practice analysis is undertaken by the panel, the competencies can be used as a source of the role analysis functions.

At a minimum, these competencies should be included as part of certification preparation courses. These courses often enroll learners who plan to take the certification exam and those new to the role and would like an orientation to the job functions.

To accomplish the synergy with the certification exam, the members of the content expert panel need to acknowledge that competencies are a major part of demonstrating the role of the NPD specialist and adopt them as part of the literature to support the role.

# Job Function Analysis

As society becomes more complex and job functions become more specialized, positions are reevaluated for appropriate title, responsibilities, and salary. Human resources departments can use the competencies as an evidence-based tool for the job analysis function.

Additionally, the person in professional development often works beyond the job requirements, putting in long hours, taking on multiple assignments, and teaching at odd hours to fulfill all roles of the NPD specialist. Using the competencies as a management tool to assign how much time or what percentage of the job should be spent on each of the key areas would be a helpful organizational tool. For this to occur, the NPD specialist will have to bring this document to the attention of human resources and managers so that an evidence-based approach can be employed to job function analysis.

# Development Plan for New Role

A very simple and logical application of the competencies is to create a development plan for a new hire into the professional development department. Ideally, those hired into the department already possess the qualifications that incorporate these factors; however, often an experienced clinician is transferred to the educator role without the necessary skills. The competencies can be used to guide both the job orientation and the staff member's development in the role while guiding the NPD specialist from novice to expert. Unit-based educators would also benefit from using a portion of the competencies to guide their movement from the clinical role into the teaching role. Facilities often hire academic educators to function in the practice development role; however, the strategies and learning outcomes used in the academic setting can be different from those in practice setting. Using the competencies to orient the academic educator will help them make a successful transition and expedite progression from novice-to-expert NPD specialist. Agreeing to meet the competencies could be a prerequisite to accepting the job role, and then strategies based on the competencies could be employed to assist in the acquisition of these skills.

# ANCC Magnet Recognition Program®

The ANCC Magnet Recognition Program® (MRP) revision in 2014 (ANCC, 2013) continues to use the Forces of Magnetism to guide its sources of evidence. There continues to be a focus on teaching and learning within MRP organizations, with a reliance upon outcomes, both process and patient, to demonstrate success with educational interventions for administrative and clinical problems. Evidence of broad participation in professional development programs remains an expectation with outcomes related to education of patients, other nurses, future nurses, and other health profession students. More important, the focus on improved patient outcomes allows for the contribution of education interventions to be used to demonstrate how clinical problems are resolved. Acknowledgment of the competencies guide the professional development role to support an evidence-based education approach to resolving practice issues.

# Need for Additional Research

Although the development and suggested applications of the competencies were based on multiple research studies, the work has just begun. Further inquiry into the role of professional development, how the practice changes over time, the importance of one function over another, and comparison to the academic and patient educator roles should be conducted.

The practice of NPD should be built upon evidence-based teaching, and we must further examine these competencies. Therefore, funded studies that look at the evidence behind practice-teaching competencies will support further development of these competencies. This requires a continued acknowledgment that practice education (professional development) is a specialty unto itself, that good clinicians can become good teachers with specialized training, and that teaching in a practice setting requires more psychomotor and affective interactions than cognitive activities.

These applications are not exhaustive but promote concrete applications for the competencies. For research to be useful, users must have a vision of what can happen as a result of the efforts. Teaching in a practice setting has a solid evidence base for job descriptions, standards, performance evaluations, development plans, and further development of standards and certification. It is the intent of this section to stimulate the reader to think of other useful applications for this work.

# References

American Nurses Association and National Nursing Staff Development Organization. (2010). *Nursing Professional Development: Scope and Standards.* Silver Spring, MD: American Nurses Publishing.

American Nurses Credentialing Center. (2013). *2014 Magnet® Recognition Program.* Silver Spring, MD: American Nurses Publishing.

National League for Nursing. (2012). *The Scope of Practice for Academic Nurse Educators.* New York: National League for Nursing.

Halstead, J. (2007). *Nurse Educator Competencies: Creating an Evidence-based Practice for Nurse Educators.* New York: National League for Nursing.

# Chapter 15

# Educational Implications of the Institute of Medicine Report

| Learning Objective |
| --- |
| **After reading this chapter the participant should be able to:** |
| ☑ Describe educational implications related to the Institute of Medicine (IOM) report, "The Future of Nursing" |

Minimum educational levels for entry into nursing practice have been debated since the 1940s, and a now infamous 1965 position paper by the American Nurses Association suggested the need for an orderly transition from hospital-based diploma nursing preparation to nursing education in colleges or universities. Now, 49 years later, despite passionate debate, increasing scope, and complexity of professional nursing role and evidence showing a link between the educational preparation of nurses and patient outcomes, little progress has been made in achieving this goal (Sigma Theta Tau International [STTI], 2011).

In October 2010, the Institute of Medicine (IOM) published *The Future of Nursing: Leading Change, Advancing Health* (IOM, 2011). This report noted that varying levels of education and competencies impede effective care for patients and promoting health. Four key messages were delivered from this report:

- Nurses should practice to the full extent of their education and training.
- Nurses should achieve higher levels of education and training through an improved education system that promotes seamless academic progression.
- Nurses should be full partners with physicians and other health professionals in redesigning healthcare in the United States.

■ Effective workforce planning and policy-making require better data collection and an improved information infrastructure.

IOM researchers identified eight recommendations (IOM, 2011):

1. Remove scope-of-practice barriers.

2. Expand opportunities for nurses to lead and diffuse collaborative improvement efforts.

3. Implement nurse residency programs.

4. Increase the proportion of nurses with a baccalaureate degree to 80% by 2020.

5. Double the number of nurses with a doctorate by 2020.

6. Ensure that nurses engage in lifelong learning.

7. Prepare and enable nurses to lead change to advance health.

8. Build an infrastructure for the collection and analysis of interprofessional healthcare workforce data.

# NPD Specialist Role in Helping Meet IOM Recommendations

The Association for Nursing Professional Development (ANPD) issued a white paper, *The Role of Nursing Professional Development in Helping Meet Institute of Medicine's Future of Nursing Recommendations* (ANPD, 2013). This paper provided specific suggestions in each of the eight major IOM recommendations for how the NPD specialist can help meet those recommendations. They used the five areas identified in the domain of responsibility in the *Nursing Professional Development: Scope and Standards of Practice* (American Nurses Association [ANA] and National Nursing Staff Development Organization [NNSDO], 2010) for the suggested activities under each of the recommendations. These are:

1. Career development responsibilities

2. Education responsibilities

3. Leadership responsibilities

4. Program management responsibilities

5. Compliance initiative responsibilities

The identified strategies were designed to demonstrate a variety of ways to help NPD specialists meet the IOM recommendations. By providing multiple strategies, NPD educators can select ones that are appropriate for their current setting and role.

The "BSN-in-10" is one strategy being suggested to help meet the IOM recommendation. The ANA House of Delegates in 2008 took the position that legislation requiring that new RNs complete the BSN within 10 years of licensure, exempting currently licensed RNs and associate degree (AD) and diploma students, is necessary to improve the quality and safety of care. Others believe that the voluntary BSN degree completion and marketplace factors will be sufficient to reach this IOM goal (Edwards, 2014).

Many institutions are implementing preferential hiring of BSN-prepared nurses. Over half of the 300 organizations that responded to a survey by the American Organization of Nurse Executives (AONE) in the fall of 2011 indicated they had such a policy. Some organization executives reported that their organizations are planning to adopt such a policy and others noted that they hire preferentially without a stated policy. Other institutions without a policy on BSN hiring are requiring that their current RN staff complete the BSN within five to six years (Edwards, 2014).

## Issues Relating to Education

Issues identified in the IOM report relating to education were availability and access to educational programs, availability of clinical sites, and financial pressures related to the cost of education. It is important to have a seamless transition between educational programs. Implications for the NPD specialist identified by Cooke (2013) included the following strategies:

- Development of academic/service partnerships
- Career counseling
- Collaboration for interprofessional, learner-directed continuing education
- Advocating for tuition reimbursement benefits
- Certification review mechanisms

Orsolini-Hain (2012) suggested that the IOM recommendation create many possibilities for community college nursing programs to be key players in ensuring that our healthcare workforce can provide accessible, high-quality healthcare for 32 million more Americans. She argued that it is time for nurse educators from all levels of education to come together for the common good and emphasized the opportunities for community college nursing programs to create new types of enduring partnerships with healthcare organizations and with our university colleagues. The author's organization helped facilitate dialogue with a community college and university that led to a special LPN-AD-BSN dual degree program for a cohort of LPNs in that organization.

A group of researchers (Spetz et al., 2014) created a dashboard to track progress toward the IOM recommendations. Their article outlined the process used to identify and develop a set of data used to track national progress toward the IOM recommendations. The data are presented in a dashboard format to visually summarize information and quickly measure progress. By identifying the indicators and the data source, this should help states and local regions in the collection of their own data.

This chapter summarized the recommendations included in the IOM *The Future of Nursing Report* and outlines implications for the NPD specialist in helping meet those recommendations. Issues related to education were also described.

# References

American Nurses Association and National Nursing Staff Development Organization. (2010). *Nursing professional development: Scope and standards of practice.* Silver Spring, MD: Nursesbooks.org.

Association for Nursing Professional Development Public Policy Committee. (2013). *ANPD White Paper: Role of nursing professional development in helping meet institute of medicine's future of nursing recommendations.* Chicago, IL: Author.

Cooke, M. (2013). Issues and trends in nursing professional development. In S.L. Bruce, (ed.), *Core curriculum for nursing professional development* (4th ed., pp. 587-613). Chicago, IL: Association for Nursing Professional Development.

Edwards, D. (2014). The marketplace speaks: Education of the nurse workforce. *Ohio Nurse, 7*(2), 1–2.

Institute of Medicine. (2011). *The future of nursing: Leading change, advancing health.* Washington, DC: National Academies Press.

Orsolini-Hain, L. (2012). The Institute of Medicine's future of nursing report: What are the implications for associate degree nursing education. *Teaching and learning in nursing, 7,* 74–77. doi: 10.1016/j.teln.2011.11.003.

Sigma Theta Tau International. (2011). *The power of ten: Nurse leaders address the profession's ten most pressing issues.* Indianapolis, IN: Author.

Spetz, J., Bates, T., Chu, L., Lin, J., Fishman, N.W., & Melichar, L. (2014). Creating a dashboard to track progress toward IOM recommendations for the future of nursing. *Policy, Politics, and Nursing Practice,* online 31 January 2014. Retrieved from *http://ppn.Sagepul.com/content/early/2014/01/29/5271544521014.* doi: 10.1177/1527154414521014.